The Orgasm Bible

Susan Crain Bakos

Author of *The Sex Bible*

The Orgasm Bible

THE LATEST RESEARCH AND TECHNIQUES
FOR REACHING MORE POWERFUL CLIMAXES MORE OFTEN

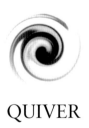

QUIVER

Text © 2008 by Susan Crain Bakos
Photography © 2008 Quiver

First published in the USA in 2008 by
Quiver, a member of
Quayside Publishing Group
100 Cummings Center
Suite 406-L
Beverly, MA 01915-6101
www.quiverbooks.com

The publisher maintains the records relating to images in this book
required by 18 USC 2257, which are located at Rockport Publishers, Inc.,
100 Cummings Center, Suite 406-L, Beverly, MA 01915-6101.

12 11 10 09 08   1 2 3 4 5

ISBN-13: 978-1-59233-281-6
ISBN-10: 1-59233-281-1

Library of Congress Cataloging-in-Publication Data

Bakos, Susan Crain.
    The orgasm bible : the latest research and techniques for reaching
  more powerful climaxes more often / Susan Crain Bakos.
            p.   cm.
Includes index.
    ISBN 1-59233-281-1
    1. Sex instruction. 2. Orgasm. I. Title.
  HQ31.B23496 2007
  613.9'6—dc22

                                        2007024802

Cover and interior design by Stephen Gleason Design

Printed and bound in Singapore

With love for Nan Wise—brilliant neuroscience researcher, compassionate therapist, very dear sister/friend

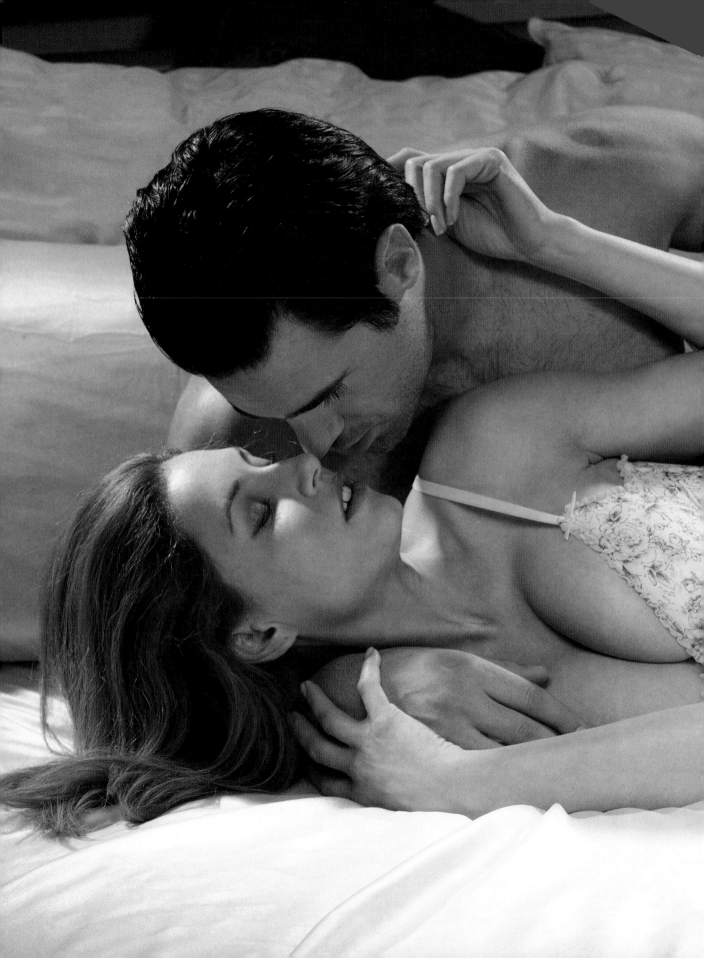

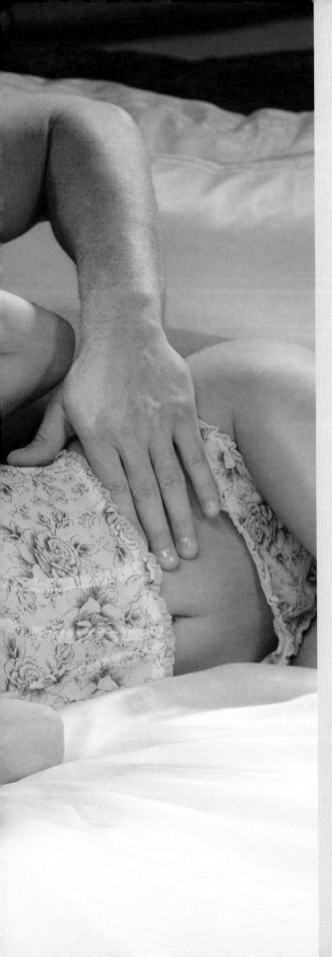

Contents

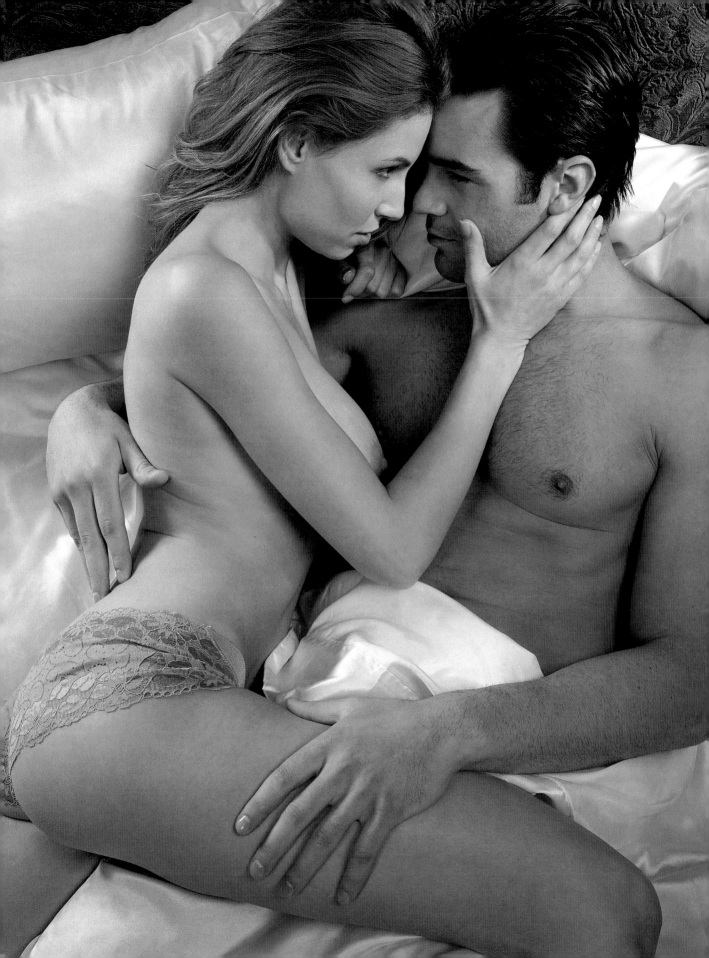

Introduction

The Hype, the Hope, the Myths, and the Truth about Orgasm

The hype, the myths, and especially the hope surrounding orgasm persist. That ballyhooed (or is it "hooey-ed"?) book *24-Hour Orgasm* was pure hype, a great cover line for selling a book. Many such cover lines have sold other books based on tiny kernels of orgasm truth exploded into nuclear popcorn—hype. The idea that love leads to orgasm: myth. Another myth: A woman can come during intercourse if a man has a big penis and knows what to do with it. You will encounter more examples of both hype and myth in the chapters that follow.

The hope? It's all a woman has if she doesn't know her own body and leaves the "job" of making orgasm happen up to her partner. Women come during passionate intercourse with no visible signs of direct clitoral stimulation in novels and mainstream movies and even in porn films where the producers and directors ought to know better. The trailer for a new adult flick by a respected woman producer shows a couple in a rear-entry intercourse position. The happy woman appears to be on the verge, but no hand is anywhere near her genitals. Now, come on! I would love to see that scene done with a finger vibe (on her finger or his) in the right place—just as I would love to see a real anal sex scene where the lube is applied copiously and the fingers, tongue, and even butt plug are introduced to relax and open the anal sphincter muscles before penetration. (Trust me: all that happens off camera now.)

You know the joke: Yes, the Prince will come—but too soon. And he will leave the Princess hanging on the edge. Why do women, and men too, put our erotic faith solely in the symbolic sword of the Prince, when women have it within their power to take themselves over the edge at any time?

We do that because generations of women and men have bought into the biggest orgasm myth of all: intimacy over orgasms. Women would rather feel close and connected to their partners than come, according to the myth. A study reported in a CNN story in November 2006 was one of many claiming that it's not orgasm but intimacy women crave. Doesn't that remind you of a woman waving away the dessert menu and saying, "Oh, no dessert for me. I shouldn't! I'll just have a bite of yours."

So women are satisfied with a bite of what he's having? The reflected glow of his orgasmic delight? Do women really not mind thrilling to his throb alone? Do men not mind the disparity?

Oh, yeah, we all mind.

Women order desserts now and still sample his. Don't you think it's time women claimed their pleasure, too?

For more than twenty years, I have been writing sex advice columns in magazines from *Penthouse Forum* to *Redbook*, and in books as well. I have surveyed and interviewed thousands of women and men. The number one question from women, both then and now, is: "How can I come during intercourse?" The number one question from men, then and now, is: "How can I give her an orgasm?"

Women mind. Men mind, too.

In fact, we mind so much that every few years major studies report great dissatisfaction in our bedrooms. Up to 70 percent of women don't reach orgasm during

"lovemaking" or "sexual encounters"—and that typically means intercourse-based sex. An equal number report loss of desire in long-term relationships, especially marriages. Men are losing desire, too.

Some studies go as far as to label women as "dysfunctional" because they don't reach orgasm and don't want sex. Is it dysfunction or a passive/aggressive rejection of the sexual status quo: He comes, she maybe does?

If women have been cheated by our reliance on the myth of intimacy over orgasm, then so have men. The pressure has been on him to do something he probably can't do no matter how "good" he is in bed: bring her to orgasm on the strength of his penis alone. That gives him "performance anxiety," his own special sex problem to complement hers.

In the 1970s, young baby boomer women gave their men a message: cunnilingus. Many got the message. Cunnilingus became not only an accepted part of sex play but also a preferred way to "give" a woman an orgasm before intercourse, where he could get his. In 2004, Ian Kerner, Ph.D., repeated the message for a new generation of men in his book *She Comes First*. In the introduction, he wrote that he was inspired to write the book by his own struggles with premature ejaculation. (His follow-up book? *He Comes Next*.)

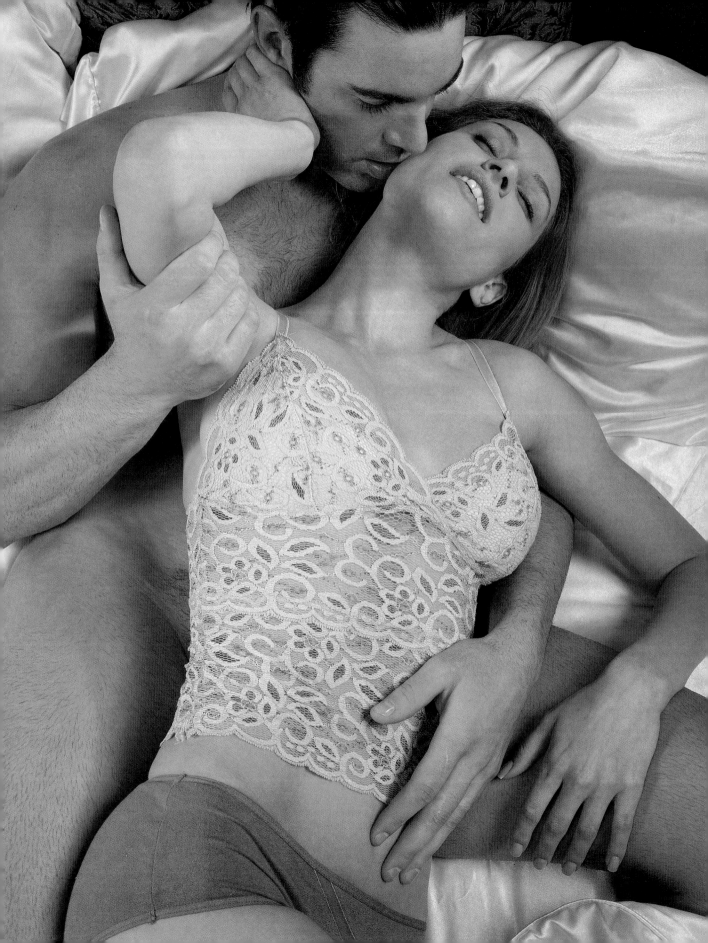

While I love Ian and his book, I wish readers could take away the wonderful information about pleasuring women without buying into the implicit premise: It really is up to him to "give" her that orgasm.

As Carlin Ross, the founder and CEO of Cherrybomb, a women's lifestyle brand, says repeatedly: "It's not his job to make her come." A feminist whose primary agenda is the sexual empowerment of women without the disenfranchisement of men, Carlin believes that "women's heads—and that includes the heads of female therapists and researchers—are so filled with guilt about sex that they perpetuate the myths in the guise of science. They bolster the belief that it is his job to make her come."

Carlin is right. From girlfriends to sex therapists to porn producers, women have all colluded to make that "his job." How much freer and more satisfying for both partners sex would be if we truly believed and accepted the immortal words of Teri Garr's character in the classic film *Tootsie*: "I [the woman] am responsible for my own orgasms!"

Orgasm is easy for men, difficult for women, the reasoning goes, yet paradoxically women can have them longer, stronger, and more often than men. Orgasm could be, should be, just as easy for women—and it would be if women embraced the orgasm truths and didn't cleave to the hype and the myths while clinging desperately to the hope. You doubt that? Consider this: Men and women reach orgasm via masturbation in about the same amount of time, five to six minutes.

That "elusive" or "problematic" female orgasm is right at her fingertips (or vibrator) when she's pleasuring herself.

The biggest truth about her orgasm is that it probably isn't going to happen via intercourse alone. Anatomy and physiology are the determining factors. Most women are not built to get all the stimulation they need to reach orgasm through the friction of intercourse. That friction works great for him. But it will only produce the same waves of ecstasy for her if she is one of approximately 25 percent of women who have what I call an "innie" clitoris. Some belly buttons pop out, some go in. Some clitorises stand out as soon as the woman is excited. Others hide beneath their hoods and the tongue must search for them, but they get what they need from intercourse friction. Intercourse alone will never do it for the woman whose clitoris is an "outie."

Nobody ever talks about this! We hide behind language that makes it sound like only a small percentage of women are "sexy" enough to come with no hands—and/or only a small percentage of men are skilled enough to bring them to orgasm with no hands. And we label women "dysfunctional" if they don't reach orgasm during intercourse alone—and, correspondingly, lose their desire for sex. How crazy is that?

Orgasms are splendid. They are worth pursuing. Having them makes everyone happier, healthier, and more connected to their own sexuality as well as to their partners. For women, the ability to reach orgasm easily and often is empowering. Yet feminists have curiously had little interest in leading women to that kind of empowerment—and have often seemed to be victims of intimacy myths themselves.

Doris Lessing was suspicious of men who were motivated to find a woman's clitoris. They "fear intimacy," she wrote. Simone de Beauvoir never had an orgasm with Jean Paul Sartre—and they call that a great love affair!—but was slavishly devoted to him, to the point of valuing his writing over her own. Both de Beauvoir and Germaine Greer held that "digital massage" of the clitoris by men "subjugated women still further." Greer encouraged women to hold out for "ecstasy" and the vaginal orgasm. American feminists of the 1970s knelt in obeisance to lesbianism but had little interest in improving sex for heterosexual women. Remember the late Andrea Dworkin's contention that all intercourse was rape?

One might think that the younger generation, especially the women—Gen X and Gen Y—have sex and orgasm figured out, but one would be wrong. *Writing in Her Way: Young Women Remake the Sexual Revolution* author Paula Kamen concluded from her interviews that twenty-something women can't tell men what they want in bed—and aren't getting it, either. Although these women lament that the men with whom they "hook up" or have "booty calls" don't care whether "we're getting off or not," they keep hooking up and answering the calls. Why? They don't want to "scare the boys away." What must the boys think of all that?

What kind of new revolution is this if the girls don't even get dinner before having sex without orgasm? What are they getting out of those hookups and booty calls? Surely not even "intimacy." The anthropologist Margaret Mead said that men and women know sexual techniques in societies where sexuality and sexual pleasure are valued. I do not recall her writing about "intimacy issues" within those societies, either.

To say that women would choose intimacy over orgasm is an insult to our intelligence anyway. How intimately connected, how close and fond does she feel lying at his side after he has come and she has not? I would wager: not very. She may even be seething with resentment. And she's certainly—according to the statistics—in no hurry to do it again. How must he feel knowing she's dissatisfied?

Men have it right: Good sex and orgasm create intimacy between lovers.

Women can have this. It's not that hard. Men want it for their partners, too.

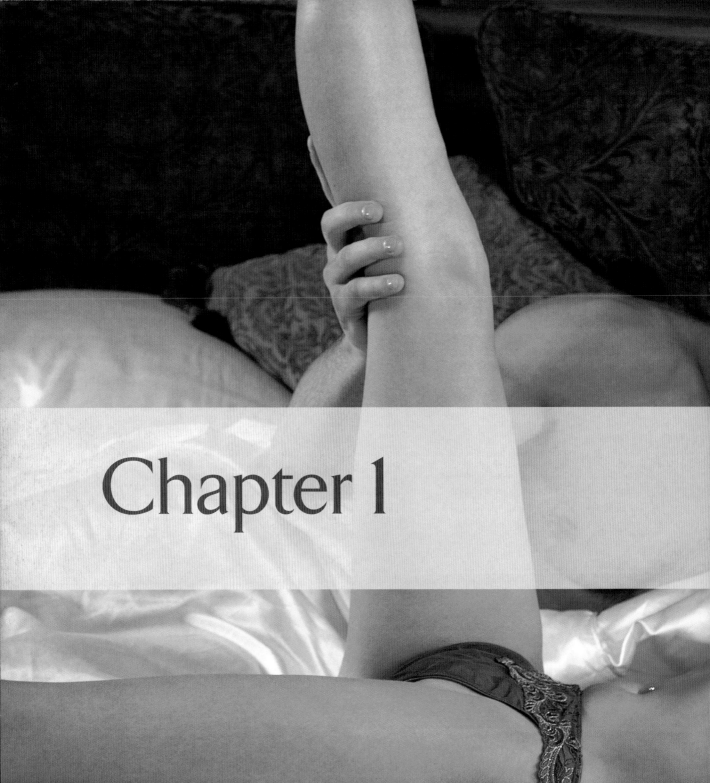

Chapter 1

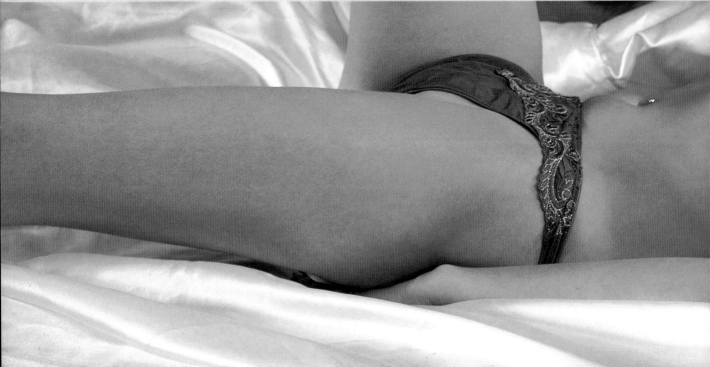

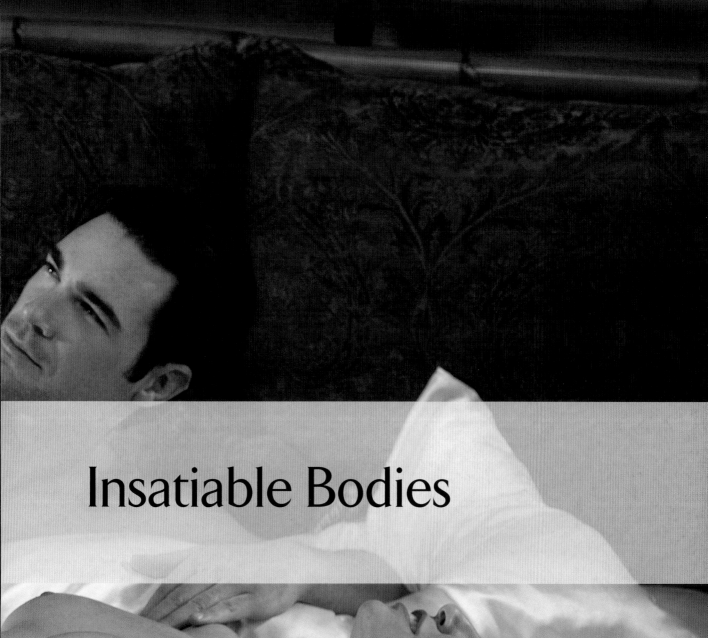

Insatiable Bodies

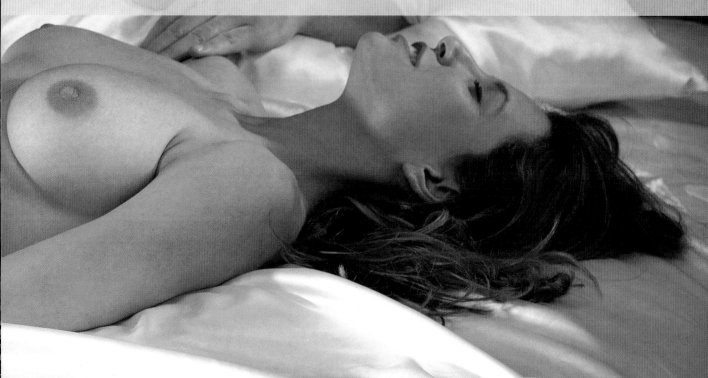

The Role of Diet and Exercise in the Lusty Life

Not only does regular, vigorous exercise improve your sex life and increase the likelihood of orgasm, but research has also shown that orgasm is beneficial to your health. And that is not exactly a new idea.

The big 1999 Chicago study, the National Health and Social Life Survey, disclosed that "sexual problems" affected 43 percent of women.

Those problems included the big three:

- Lack of desire

- Difficulty in becoming aroused

- Inability to reach orgasm

Research conducted at the University of Texas in Austin, however, found that women with low sexual arousal who did twenty minutes of aerobic exercise, such as fast walking, jogging, or riding a stationery bike, increased their level of arousal and desire.

Regular exercise is just as important in maintaining his lusty life as hers. In fact, as men age past forty, they need to maintain their body to sustain their penis. Excessive drinking and smoking, weight problems, and hypertension put weights on the end of the penis, bringing it down. Viagra and Cialis can help, but they leave a telltale flush on your face—and nothing beats a natural high, anyway.

The History of Hysteria

Doctors from Hippocrates to Freud preached the power of orgasm and sometimes stimulated orgasm in their female patients to "cure" a range of ills, most often one called "hysteria." In ancient Egypt and Greece, they thought hysteria was caused by sexual deprivation, but they didn't look to doctors to cure it.

The vibrator was actually introduced in the 1880s as a medical device for treating hysterical women via genital massage, relieving doctors of the difficult work of doing that by hand. If you've ever wondered why so many female characters in Victorian novels were prone to hysteria, now you know.

As psychology became a prominent discipline, "hysteria" morphed into "frigidity" and then "female sexual dysfunction," or FSD. Numerous studies in recent years have reported large numbers of dysfunctional women.

Regular stretching makes your movements more sensuous and fluid.

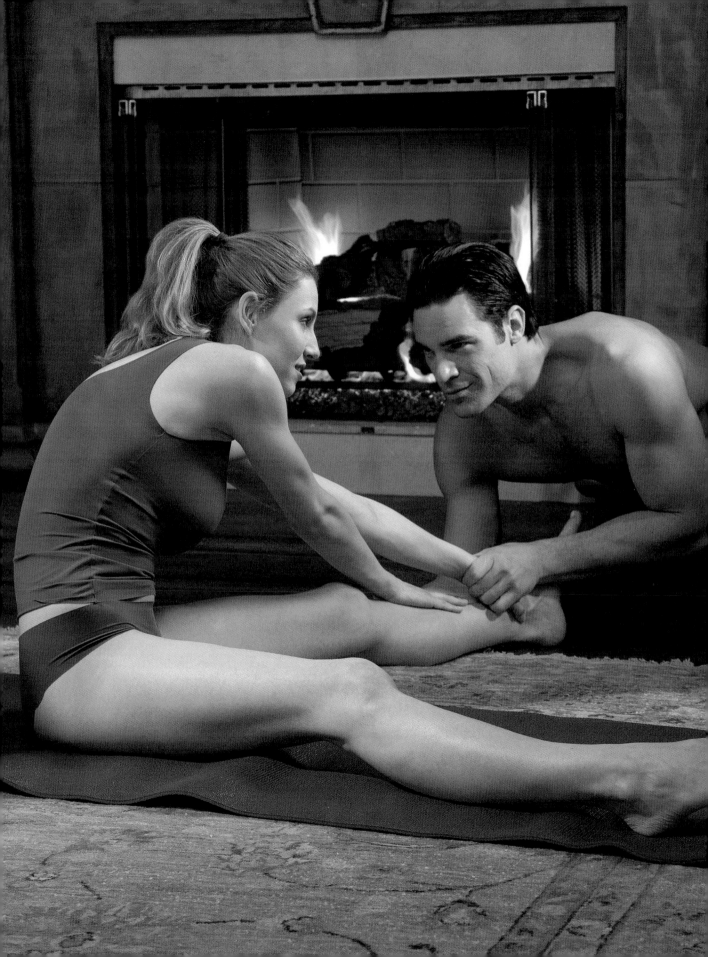

Orgasm and Your Health

Hundreds of research studies have concluded that orgasm is beneficial to health.

Here are a few highlights:

- A U.S. research study on middle-aged men suggested a relationship between the levels of sex hormones in the body and a reduction in the risk of heart disease.

- An Israeli study found similar results for middle-aged women.

- Some studies recently have suggested that oxytocin, a sex chemical, may play a preventive role in breast cancer.

- A U.S. study found that women who had orgasms before sleep reported 57 percent fewer sleep problems than women who didn't.

- Many studies around the world have reported on the power of orgasm to alleviate pain.

Passion Killers

Keep in mind that the following will kill your passion—and that of your partner:

- Excessive eating

- Excessive drinking

- Smoking

- Drugs, both recreational and some prescription drugs, especially antidepressants and medications for high blood pressure

- Obesity

- Lack of attention to appearance and grooming

TIP

Yoga is great for stretching, relaxing, and getting in touch with your sexuality. Consider taking a yoga class with your partner. Or buy a simple beginner's guide book. Practice positions facing one another or side-by-side. If you prefer more high energy workouts yet don't want to compete in games like tennis, then jog or speed walk together—and talk along the way about what you want to do in bed later.

Exercising together will give you heightened awareness of your partner's body.

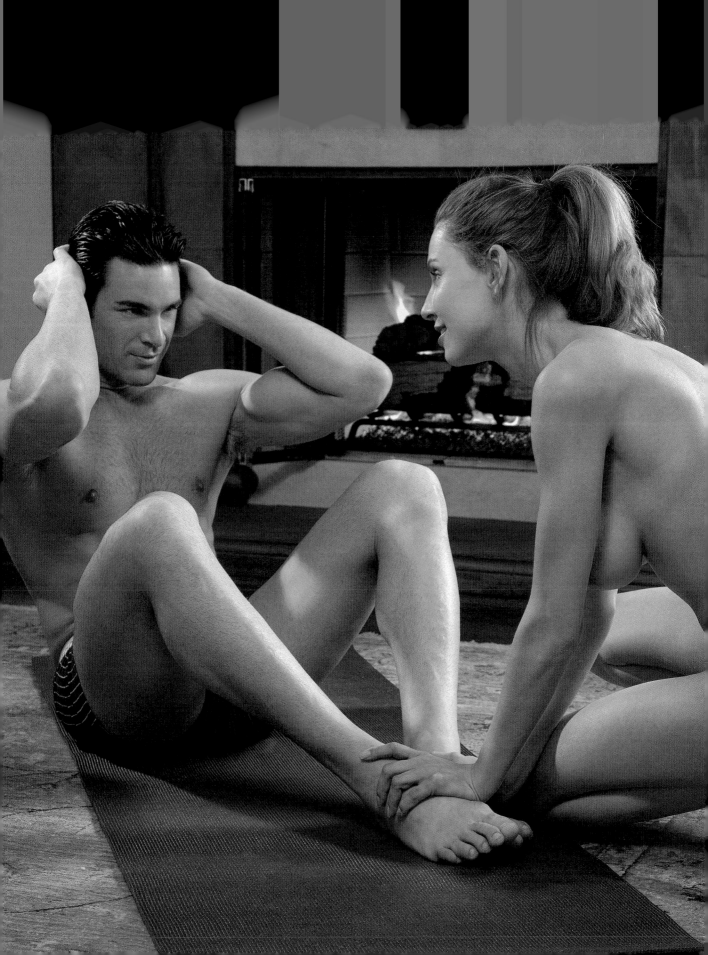

The Indispensable Exercise: Kegels

You cannot have a great sex life with a flaccid pubococcygeus (PC) muscle. It's just not possible. You won't be able to grasp his penis as tightly as you'd like when he's inside you. You won't have the ability to make your orgasm come on faster, longer, and stronger. Without exercising this critical muscle after childbirth, you will never regain sexual tone. (And do you think so many women would need adult diapers if they had a stronger PC?)

Don't skip this section. Do your Kegels. It's critical to your sex life and just not that hard to do. Standing in line, driving, working out, reading a book, watching TV—Kegel time, any time. And yes, he needs to have a strong PC muscle too to sustain intercourse longer and have some control over his ejaculation.

Here's how: The PC muscle is a hammock-like muscle that stretches from the pubic bone to the coccyx (tailbone) in both sexes. It forms the floor of your pelvic cavity. Locate your PC muscle by stopping and starting the flow of urine. After you have found the PC muscle, start with a short Kegel sequence, and then add a long Kegel sequence.

Short Kegel Sequence

Contract the muscle 20 times at approximately one squeeze per second. Exhale gently as you tighten only the muscles around your genitals (including the anus), but not the muscles in your buttocks. Don't bear down when you release. Simply let go.

Do two sets of 20 twice a day. Gradually build up to two sets of 75 per day.

Long Kegel Sequence

Hold the muscle contractions for a count of three. Relax between contractions. Work up to holding for ten seconds, then relaxing for ten seconds. Again start with two sets of 20 and build up to two sets of 75.

Once you are doing 300 contractions a day of the combined short and long sequences, you will be ready to add the push-out.

The Push-Out

After releasing the contraction, push down and out gently, as if you were having a bowel movement with your PC muscle. I said gently. It's a slow release of that muscle, with some light pressure exerted while pushing down (out).

Once you've mastered the push-out, create Kegel sequences that combine long and short repetitions with push-outs. After six weeks of daily sets of 300, you should have a well-developed PC muscle and can keep it that way by doing sets of 150 several times a week.

Kegel Exercisers

Kegel exercisers, such as Candida Royalle's little barbell, can add fun to the routine. You simply pull the bar into your vagina using your PC muscle, and then expel it the same way. Pull in, push out. Easy. Now try it with a vibe and then a penis.

"Clearly orgasm represents a lot more than the few moments of neuropsychological release by which it's clinically defined... orgasm both gratifies and confounds us in ways that transcend our biology."

—Nina Hartley, *Nina Hartley's Guide to Total Sex*

For Her: The Shag Workout

The Shag Workout is specifically designed to boost your sexual energy and enhance your orgasms as you're toning and trimming. A three-stage workout that aims to develop flexibility in the pelvic area and increase sexual confidence, energy, and libido while improving general fitness, the Shag is essentially an aerobic workout with a lot of focus on the pelvic region. The extra ingredient: sexual meditation. Created by Gymbox in London, the Shag is intense but easy to learn and aims to make you F.A.S.T.E.R. (Flexibility, Agility, Stamina, Tone, Endurance, and Rhythm).

Step #1: Increase Pelvic Flexibility and Heighten Erotic Awareness

Warm-up: Start with your favorite aerobic activity, for example jazz dancing, cycling, or running on the treadmill, and do it for 10 minutes. While you're exercising, practice creative visualization. Think hot. Fantasize an erotic encounter or simply concentrate on focusing sexual energy to your genitals.

Step #2: Intensify and Add Pelvic Techniques

Kick into erotic/aerobic higher gear by adding the following:

The Hot Hips Swivel: After your brief warm-up, stand with your feet about 2 feet apart, with your knees slightly bent and your lower tummy slightly protruding. Put your hands on your waist. Imagine a cone of erotic fire with the tip at your navel spreading throughout your pelvic region. Swivel your hips to the right, front, left, and back in a counterclockwise direction. Work those hips! Inhale and contract your PC muscles as you move your hips forward. Exhale and release as you move them backward. Move in a dozen smooth, continuous circles. Then reverse direction and do a dozen clockwise swivels.

Now add:

The Lusty Cat: Get down on all fours. Lean forward with most of your weight on your arms and your butt in the air. Rock your pelvis only (either side-to-side or front-to-back) for 1 to 3 minutes. Then begin to move slowly across the room like a cat in heat, keeping your belly low but not touching the floor. As you move forward, lower your head close to the floor and make the motion a cat makes licking up spilled milk, with your head down, then come up slowly. This loosens tense muscles in your neck and shoulders and allows the sexual energy to flow up and down your spine. Squeeze your PC muscle and inhale on the downward movement, then release your PC muscle and exhale on the upward movement. Move fast, then slow, flexing your PC muscle and breathing in time. Do this for 3 to 5 minutes.

> ## REAL TALK
>
> "My walk is more sensual, freer, and looser, and so is the way I move in bed. I didn't realize how much tension I held in that part of my body until I started doing this routine."
>
> **—Jennie, 37**

Pelvic twists strengthen your PC muscle and open up your body for more intense orgasms.

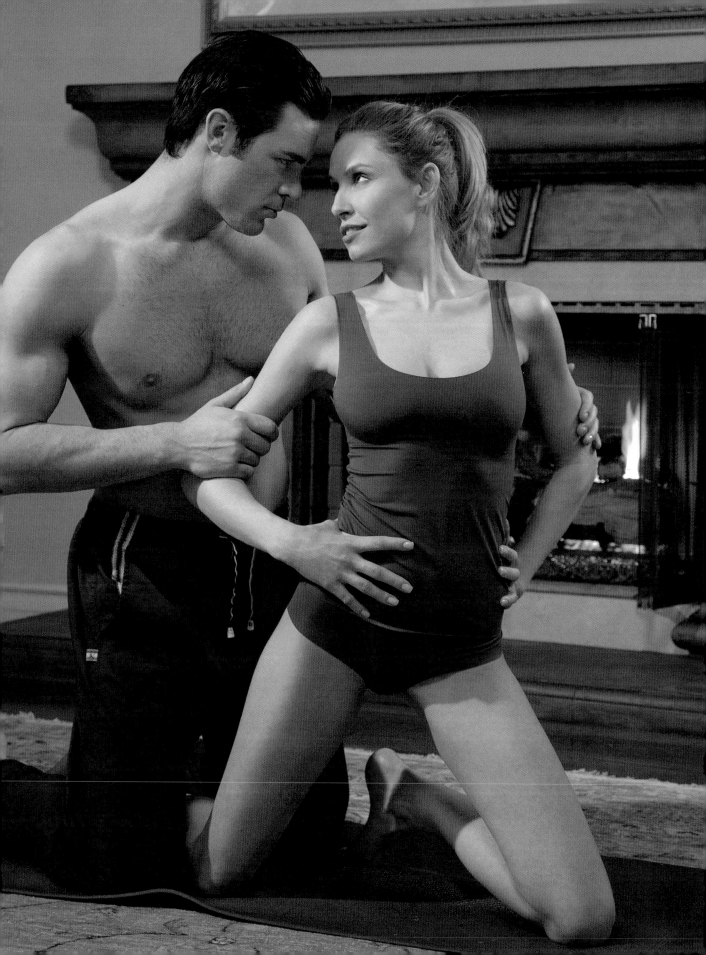

Step #3: Increase Sexual Confidence

With this exercise, you will feel sexually alive and more aware of your body, and the feeling will carry over long after the workout. Like other yoga exercises, the Lusty Cat releases energy in a way that reduces tension. The following move specifically combines tension reduction with PC work.

The Hungry Lioness: Get down on all fours. Lean forward with your chest near but not on the floor and your butt in the air. Start a vigorous back-and-forth rocking motion with your pelvis as you keep your chest and back relaxed. The rocking takes place in your pelvis only! Do this for 1 to 3 minutes. Then relax the pelvic muscles and thrust your body forward, with your weight on your arms, like a hungry lioness sensing the presence of her mate. As you lean forward, inhale and gently squeeze your buttocks together. Now push your body back, reapportioning your weight more on your knees than on your arms. As you exhale, relax your pelvis and buttocks. Repeat the movements for another minute or two.

Step #4: Increase Your Sexual Energy and Libido

Move back into an aerobic routine like kick-dancing (see below). Regular dancing, even for 10 or 15 minutes two or three times a week, increases your interest in sex while giving you a good cardio workout.

Kick-dancing: Dance to the music and in the style of your choice, but add kicks, kicking as high and as often as you can. Jazz dancing is good, too. If you're new to dance, start with modest kicks and build up slowly to avoid injury. Do this for at least 5 minutes, building up to 15 minutes on days you have time for a longer workout.

Step #5: Reith Tantra

Use your "winding down" time—and take advantage of all that released sexual energy—to learn a new sexual technique, such as spreading or "expanding" your orgasm.

Expanding orgasm: Masturbate using a vibrator or your hand. As soon as you become highly aroused, use your other hand to massage the area of your vulva, inner thighs, and groin with light, shallow strokes. Tell yourself that you are spreading arousal throughout your genitals and entire pelvic region. Continue massaging during your orgasm, imagining that you are spreading the orgasm into your whole body. After orgasm, continue stimulating your genitals. You will feel the orgasm continue to spread, and you will probably have another or several orgasms, perhaps smaller ones that feel like aftershocks. Some women report actually feeling the orgasm from the top of their heads to the soles of their feet.

Step #6: Meditate

That's sexual meditation. Close your eyes. Breathe deeply and slowly. As you breathe, focus your mind on the sexual experience you've just had. Now put your man into the picture. Imagine yourself practicing this new technique with him tonight.

Rocking the hips in The Hungry Lioness position sexually charges the pelvic area.

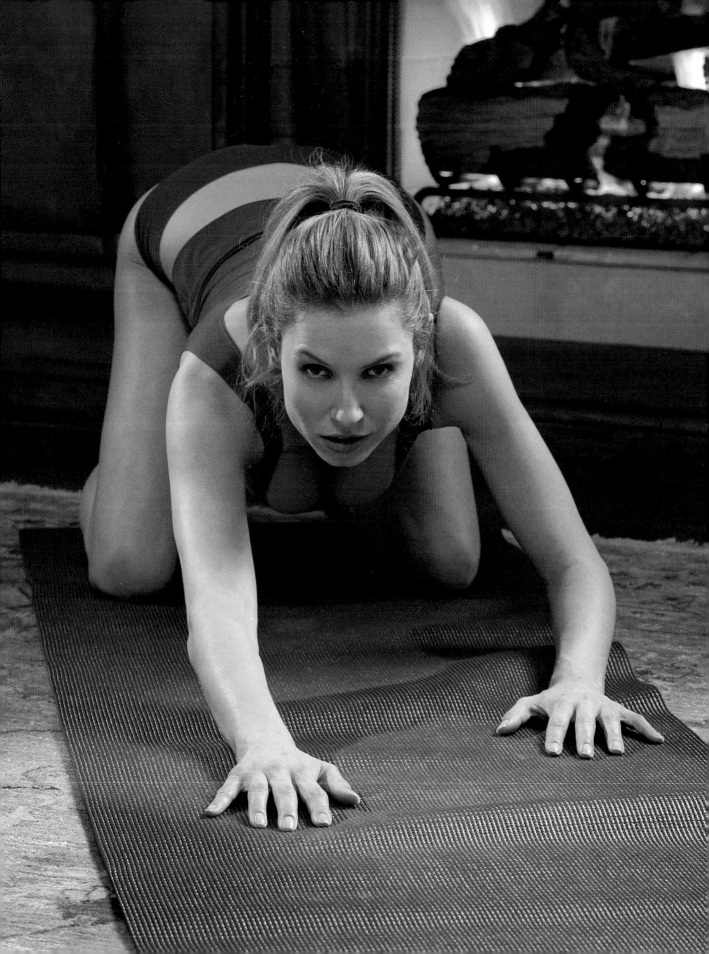

For Both of You: Kundalini Yoga

Kundalini is an area of sexual energy within your body. It is often symbolized by a serpent coiled into three and a half circles with its tail in its mouth. Some experts have told me that it sits in your back, in an inverted triangle below your waist with the tip resting above your tailbone. Others have said that the seat of Kundalini is the navel chakra, a place beginning two to three inches below the belly button and ending above the genitals. As any true Yogi master would say: Experience it for yourself. Whether you feel it sitting in your back or your belly, focus on unfurling and spreading that energy into your genitals. Your Kundalini and your PC muscle will take you places you didn't think you could go.

Unlike other forms of yoga, Kundalini does not require that you assume defined poses. Start in a simple yoga pose, standing with your feet apart, knees slightly bent, and eyes down.

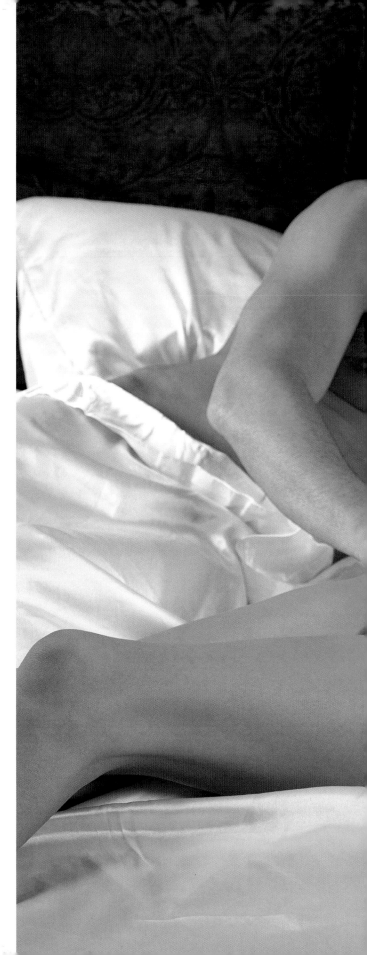

Stroke your partner's pelvic area gently but firmly to open up the navel chakra and stimulate the sexual power center.

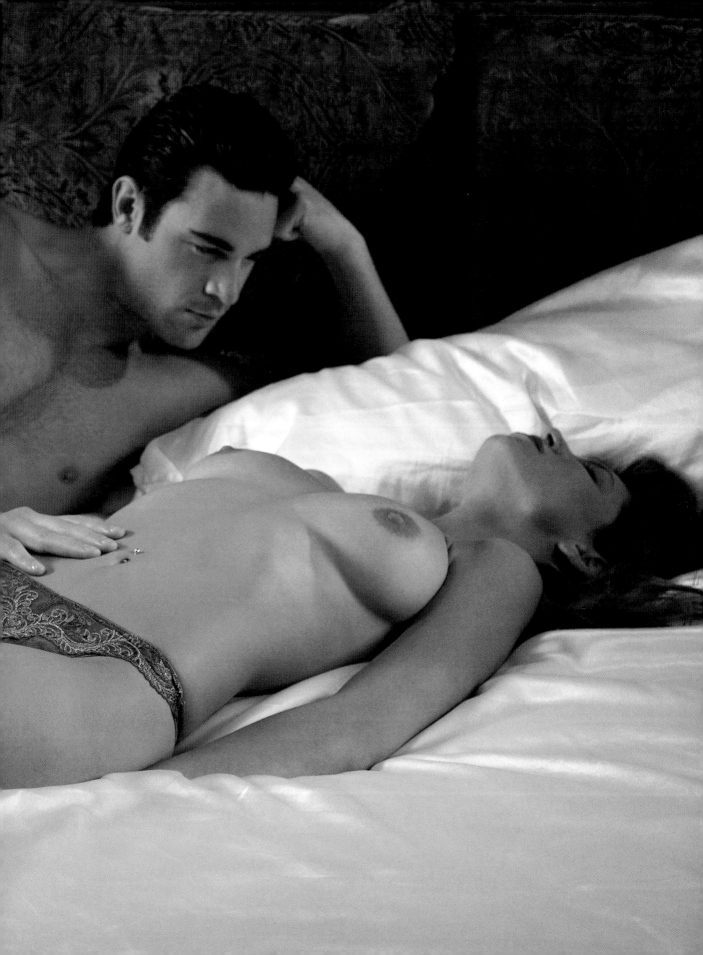

Freeing the Kundalini Energy: Exhale deeply. Imagine yourself collapsing more deeply into your Kundalini seat with each exhalation. Close your eyes. As you inhale slowly, raise your head, and feel the Kundalini energy rising. Let your hands float at your sides. Now, exhale, letting your head come down again. As you continue breathing, let your body move any way it wants to move. Feel the energy and flow with it.

Do the Freeing the Kundalini Energy exercise side-by-side or facing one another. Now, go through some easy couple's yoga exercises that will sexually energize you together.

Connecting Energies: Facing each other, with knees bent, make eye contact, and breathe together, inhaling and exhaling in time. Open up your arms and hold them around your partner, first without touching. Then hold your partner loosely by the shoulders, and breathe together for a few minutes. Feel the sexual energy pulsating throughout one body and into the other.

Rising Energies: Facing each other at arm's length apart, hold hands. Bounce gently together. Then slowly squat down to the floor. Resting on the balls of your feet, rock gently, lending each other support through clasped hands. Feel the Kundalini energy uncoiling inside your bodies. Now slowly rise together. As you rise, the Kundalini rises inside each of you. Repeat the squatting and rising, moving rhythmically. After a few times, focus on coordinating your breathing. Repeat several times.

TIP

If you want to study Kundalini in greater depth, find a teacher or a class rather than relying on a book alone. The discipline combines physical and mental exercises to connect body and mind. The basic techniques are cross-legged positions, strict positioning of the spine (usually upright), erotic use of breath, and mental focus (often on breathing or a mantra—a word used in meditation).

Studies have shown that regular practice of Kundalini can lower blood pressure, regulate heart rate, and aide in muscle relaxation. Some therapists include yoga, often Kundalini specifically, in their treatment of clients, particularly those suffering from obsessive-compulsive disorder (OCD).

Breathe together for a few minutes. Lightly touch each other to feel the sexual energy pulsating from one body to another.

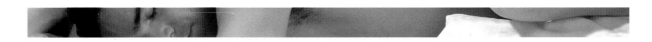

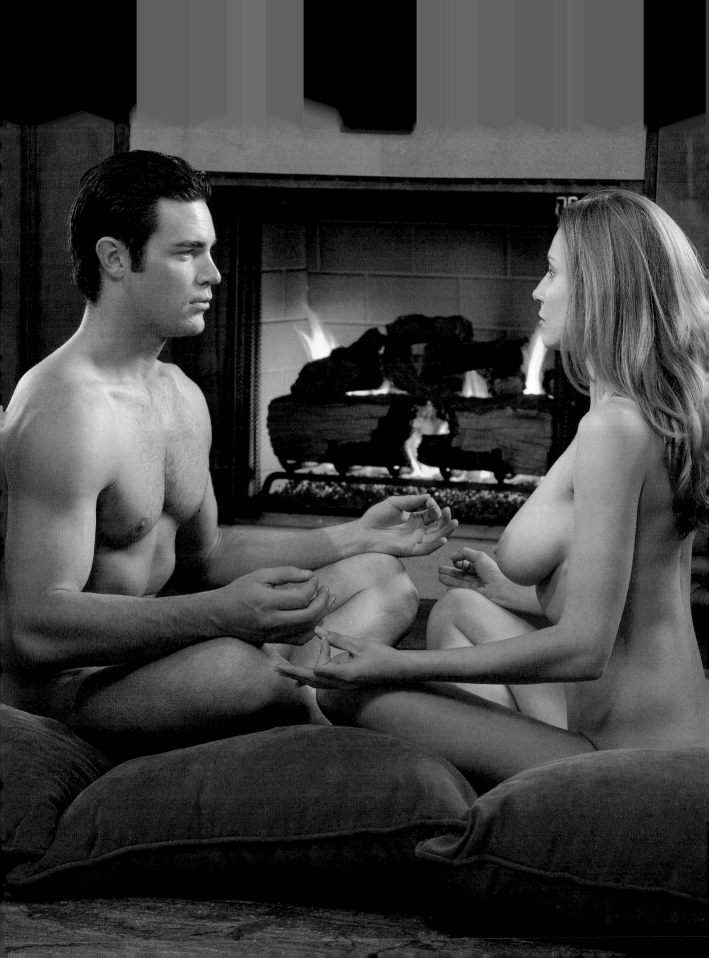

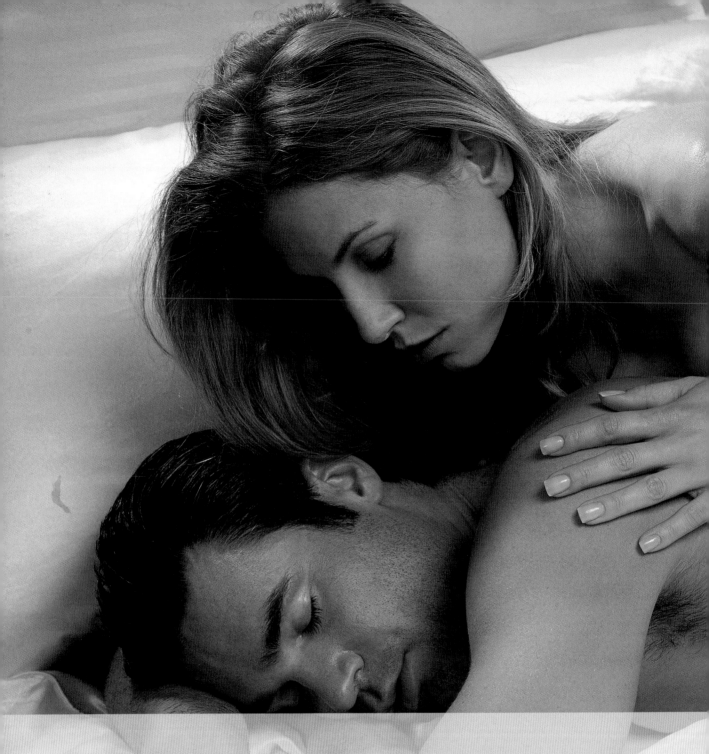

Chapter 2

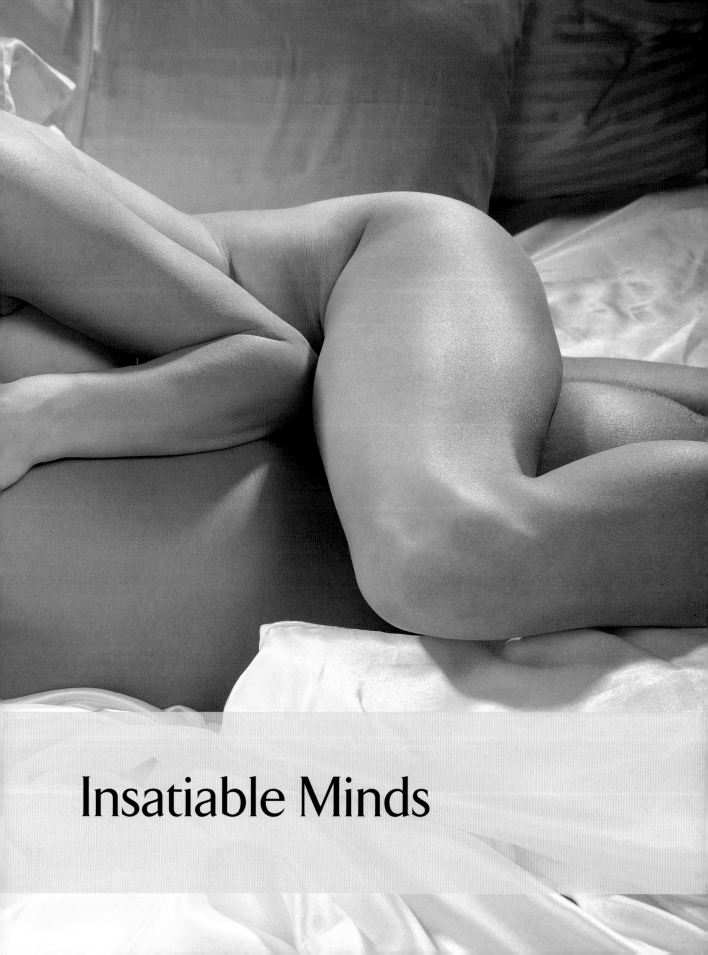

Insatiable Minds

Sex begins in the head—both in the brain and in the mind. Erotic longing, that desire we feel for one another, triggers arousal. And let's be honest: Desire is stronger early in the relationship than it is after familiarity sets in. If you can't sustain it by frequent separations or reignite it by adding "taboo" elements such as discreet cheating or mutually sanctioned affairs, one-night stands, or polyamorous liaisons, then you absolutely must heat things up through fantasy and by learning new techniques and trying new positions.

You need to keep that mind/brain-to-genital connection snapping like a hot wire in a rainstorm—at least a good part of the time. And here's something that short-circuits the connection: Women will lose their arousal if they catch a glimpse of their ass dimples in the mirror while they're having sex. A woman's body image issues often hold her back. That just doesn't happen to men. Men are never thinking, "Do my thighs look flabby in this position?"

You have to trust me on this: If a man is naked in your bed, then he isn't repulsed by your body. He has a wonderful ability to focus on the parts he likes and let the rest ease into soft focus. And his erection, the sweat on his brow, and the look of lust in his eyes are sure indicators that he has found something he likes.

Her Insatiable Mind

Women generally claim that they think about sex and fantasize less than men do. Partly, that's a denial issue. Being less obviously connected to their genitals, and thus their arousal, women dismiss or negate sexual thoughts and fantasies. Some women just don't recognize that they're thinking about sex when they are!

You doubt me? Research scientists, including Barry Komisaruk, Carlos Beyer-Flores, and Beverly Whipple, authors of the recent and acclaimed *The Science of Orgasm*, have proved it in the lab. Women attached to electrodes measuring arousal and women participating in brain scan research often show signs of arousal while watching explicit erotic material—while they are claiming, "No, I'm not turned on."

Old stereotypes die hard even in new generations. Are we passing this stuff down in the breast milk?

In days past, female fantasies had to be obsessively "romantic" to be acceptable. The danger there? The fantasy stopped before the sex really began and women had even more reason to equate lust with love. But Nancy Friday's 1991 book on women's fantasies, *Women On Top*, brought the female fantasy out of the closet. The women she interviewed fantasized about S/M, bondage, group sex, rape, and multiple partners. They were just as kinky as their men.

And here is a new trend: Women under forty have more girl-on-girl fantasies, with women under thirty reporting that as their number one fantasy on sites like Cherrybomb and in magazine surveys.

According to a 2006 article in the *Journal of Sex Research*, Australian researchers studied 19,000 people and discovered that 76 percent of women who slept with another woman reached orgasm, compared to only 59 percent of women who slept with men. London's *Daily Mail* reported this story under the headline: "Lesbians have more orgasms." And many studies put the number of orgasmic women sleeping with men somewhat lower than that.

Sexual fantasy builds anticipation and puts you in touch with your body's unique sexual responses.

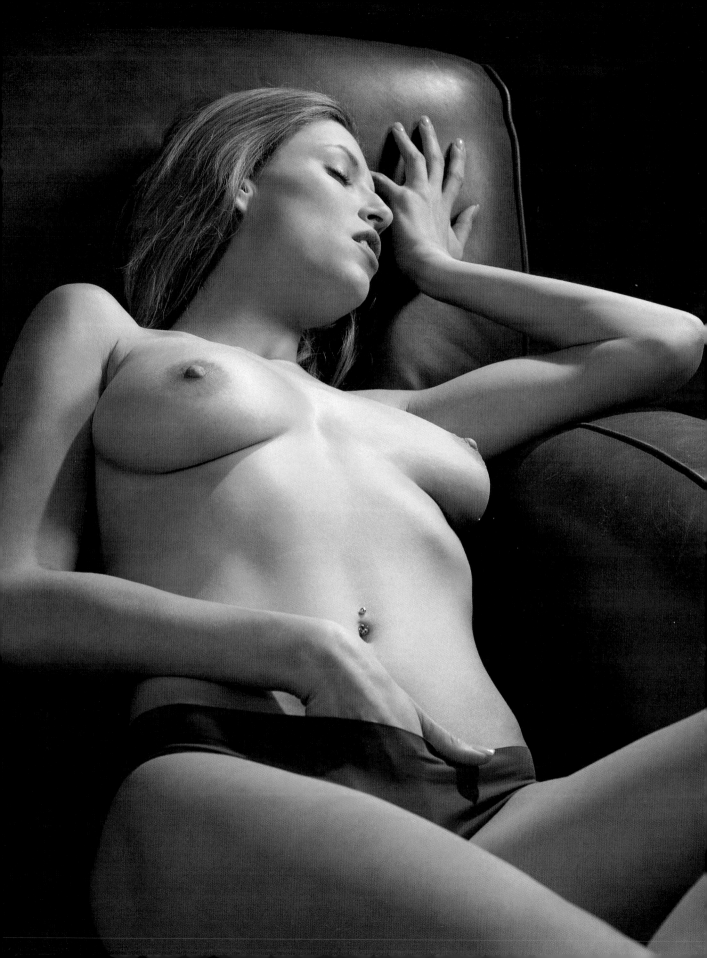

Nurture Your Fantasies

A rich fantasy life is fertile ground for sex. Here are some things you can do:

- Read, whether it's erotic, mainstream, or X-rated.

- Watch films with erotic content.

- Keep a sex journal, recording random randy thoughts, comments on your sex life, and inspirational quotes. (You can do this on the computer, but there is something very sensually satisfying about buying a beautiful book and actually putting pen to paper.) Paste in photos of sexy men and snippets of erotic art.

- Experiment with fantasies, especially while masturbating. Nothing is taboo.

- Encourage him to trigger your fantasies through voice, text, and e-mail messages.

- Get to know your "favorite friend," the fantasy that arouses you no matter what.

"Some women can think themselves off—an awesome accomplishment. They become so intensely aroused fantasizing sex that they orgasm, usually aided by flexing their PC muscles. When men do something like this, it is called premature ejaculation and it is not awesome."

—Dr. Barry Komisaruk, *The Science of Orgasm*

Sex and Relationships

When the results of a German study on female sexual attitudes and behaviors was released in late 2006, many were shocked to read this finding: Women lose more interest in sex once they feel secure in a relationship than men do! So much for the comfortable theory that a woman only opens up sexually when she feels emotionally secure.

REAL TALK

Why girl—on—girl?

"Women get disappointed in men. I started having sex with my girl roommate after we both broke up with boyfriends. We were 26 and 27. The sex was okay, but we were missing 'the dick,' so we started running ads on Craigslist for a male partner to join us. The threesomes were hot. Then I met a new guy. She's with another girl."

—Lisa, 30

———•———

"Playing with girlfriends doesn't feel like cheating on your man. I had my first oral orgasm with a girlfriend. Even if your guy finds out you're playing around with a girlfriend, he doesn't really care. It turns him on."

—Jennie, 25

Experiment with different sexual fantasies. For example, role-play a sexy tryst between assistant and boss and flip the gender roles.

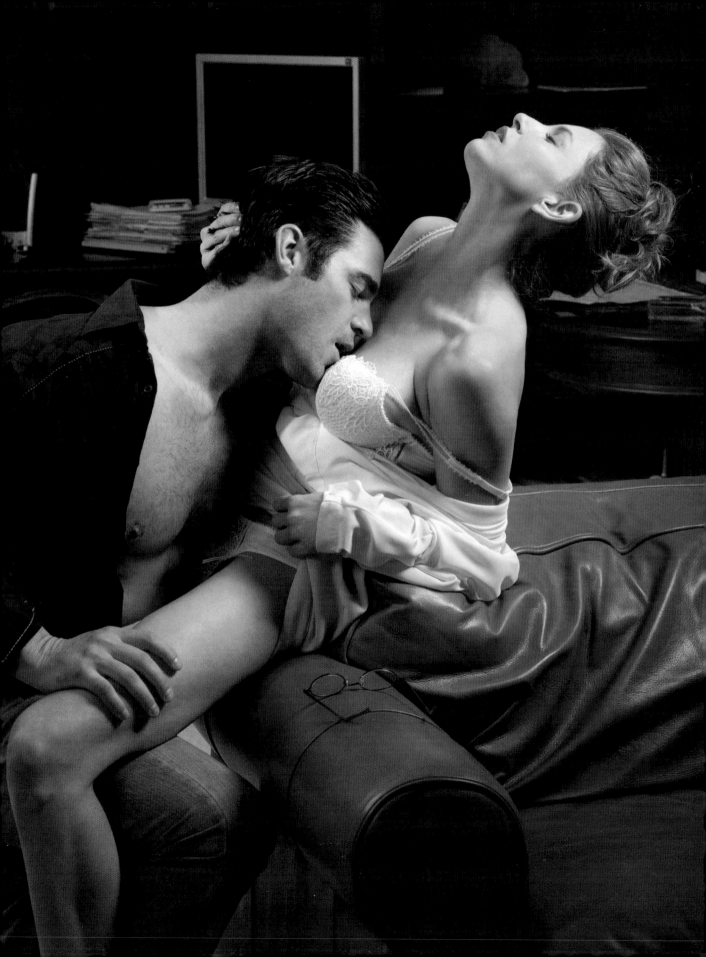

Think Yourself Off

Gina Ogden, Ph.D., author of the classic *Women Who Love Sex*, found that some women—call them lucky or "hypersexed"—can reach orgasm via extra genital stimulation alone, such as having their breasts sucked or their inner thighs kissed. Even fewer can "think off" or reach orgasm via fantasy alone.

At one time, Annie Sprinkle, author/sexpert/performance artist/goddess guide, taught workshops in "thinking off," a skill most women will not master. However, translating her techniques to lovemaking will encourage a sexual mind-set and help women be more orgasmic with their partners.

1. Establish an erotic mood with candles, wine, sexy clothing, or music—whatever does it for you.

2. Create a lush, passionate fantasy—and make it graphic.

3. Take a dozen deep breaths, then a dozen shallow ones. Use your breath to create physical desire. (Also try adding the techniques for The Orgasm Loop discussed in Chapter 11.)

4. Flex your PC muscles in time with your panting.

If you don't manage to reach orgasm through breathing and flexing, then just use your hand or vibrator to get there.

Women who put sex at or near the top of their "To Think" list are women who consistently reach orgasm. Every time you brush aside a sexy thought or an erotic fantasy, you are saying: I don't have time for my own pleasure. And that's a bad message to keep giving yourself. Indulge your sexy brain. Think, and you will come.

REAL TALK

How do you get your guy to fantasize about you?

"I send him graphic text messages. But I am prepared to follow through on the promises."
—Kelli, 26

—— • ——

"Leave him with a sense memory—your fragrance lingering on his sheets, a bit of lipstick on his collar, a little bruise or indentation from your fingernail where you gripped his ass so hard while you were coming."
—Gina, 42

—— • ——

"You keep surprising him! He's given up on getting anal sex from you and then you buy the butt plug and lube. Or you rent the really dirty porn flick."
—Christine, 38

His Insatiable Mind

According to some studies, men think about sex as often as every eleven seconds—and the younger the man, the more often it is. Men are much more willing to acknowledge that the fleeting admiration of an attractive person is a sexual thought. Men think: I'd love to have those legs wrapped around my neck. Women think: What a nice tie he's wearing.

Men do not censor their erotic thoughts. If they are smart, they don't share most of them with their girlfriends or wives. They merely delight in them in private.

Women could learn a lot from men.

Fantasy is a nearly universal experience, a mental aphrodisiac with amazing powers. Sometimes it is a conscious process, sometimes not. But if you are not satisfied with your sex life and you aren't using fantasy to create and sustain arousal, you are missing something.

His Fantasies and What They Mean

He is most likely to fantasize:

- Something kinky—bondage, S/M, coming on your face, or even worse things he's seen on the Internet, such as a hundred men coming on someone's face

- Sex with your mother, sister, best friend, or Gwen Stefani

- Sex with your mother, sister, best friend, or Gwen Stefani—and you

- Sex acts disconnected from the rest of the body, such as a porn close-up shot of a blow job or anal sex

- Anal sex with you, like they do it in the porn movies where the guy just "slips it in"

And that means what? Only that he has an active fantasy life. And, yes, he might do some of those things if you'd let him—but probably not sex with your mother unless she is Goldie Hawn. Unless he has nothing but violent fantasies and can't be aroused without them, then he's "normal"—whatever that means.

TIP

———•———

If you need help fantasizing, consider viewing some erotic images. Doing so—and acknowledging your subsequent arousal—may be key in getting you pumped up for the big event.

And ladies: don't think viewing erotic images only works for men. A 2006 study focused on arousal in male and female brains conducted at Washington University in St. Louis (U.S.) revealed a surprising find: Women registered erotic images in the brain more quickly than men. The men, however, acknowledged that the images aroused them, while most women denied they were aroused, or, in many cases, even claimed they did not recall the images. (Ladies, the brain activity says otherwise.)

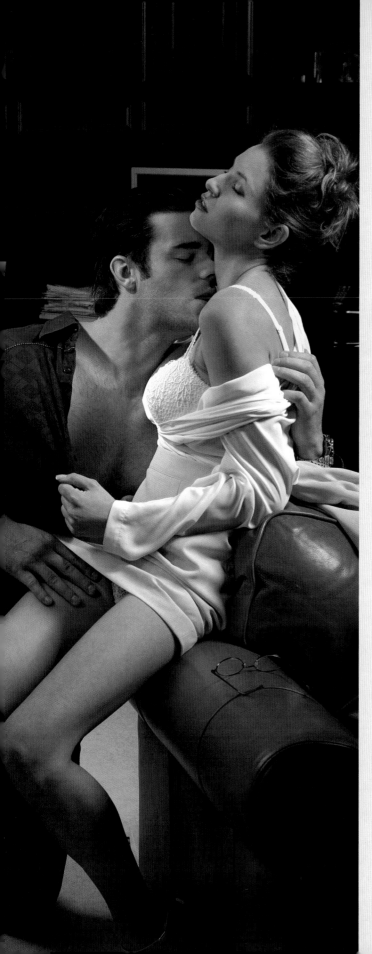

What fantasy encounters worked for you?

"I was the boss and he was the assistant. We both wore white shirts and ties, but he was naked from the waist down while I had on a thong, stockings, and stilettos. I made him get down on his knees and eat me out. It was hot."
—Jasmine, 25

——— . ———

"We took turns being master/mistress and slave. I didn't want to be the slave but she wouldn't do it if I wouldn't, so I did. I was shocked at how much I liked being told to lick her boots and getting my ass paddled."
—John, 40

——— . ———

"I wore a baby-blue bridesmaid's dress with a tiara and pretended I was Cinderella and he had to be the Prince and make me come. Very corny, but fun. My Cinderella was a dirty girl who needed a lot more than a kiss on the mouth— and she turned out to be a bit of a dom."
—Rebecca, 31

Make your fantasy role playing hot. Write the script together before your encounter and tell your partner exactly where to touch you.

Couple Fantasy Encounters

Carol Pasahow, Ph.D., developed a program specifically for her clients who said they had no time for sex. Based on quickies and fantasy encounters, the program has been successful not only with her clients but also with couples I've interviewed who learned how to do it from her book, *Sexy Encounters*. By creating a fantasy and writing its script together, the couple starts thinking more, and more creatively, about sex.

Here's how to have a fantasy encounter as a one-week adventure:

1. On the first night, talk about fantasy scenarios and select one that you both find arousing.

2. On days two through six, e-mail one another with ideas for the plot, and then take a little time each night before you go to bed to write your script together. Write erotic and descriptive dialogue, such as "The curve of your hips in the candlelight was like a sensuous sliver of the moon in the sky." Don't be afraid to go over the top.

3. Assemble props—like masks, costumes, sex toys—ahead of time. This is a great time to play with edible body paints.

4. Act out your script as if you were presenting an erotic play (such as a boss/assistant fantasy).

Keep in mind that your fantasy scenario is probably not one of the fantasies that gets you off in private. So, don't try to force or coerce your partner into buying into your scenario. The key is choosing a fantasy that will arouse both of you.

Keep a few myths and misinformation about fantasy encounters in mind. Remember, these are *not* true!

- It's always good to share your fantasies.

- Fantasizing during lovemaking means you are bored with your partner.

- Acting out a favorite fantasy will always be as hot as you dreamed it would be.

- Fantasizing about another partner is cheating.

- If you fantasize it, you want to do it, whether that's rape, a homosexual encounter, group sex—whatever.

"So much of sex is in the head that we can ruin a good experience by letting negative thoughts intrude before we're fully aroused. Try thinking, YES instead of NO, I WANT, not I'M NOT IN THE MOOD—and your body will follow your mind."

—**Nan Wise**, "The Love Coach"

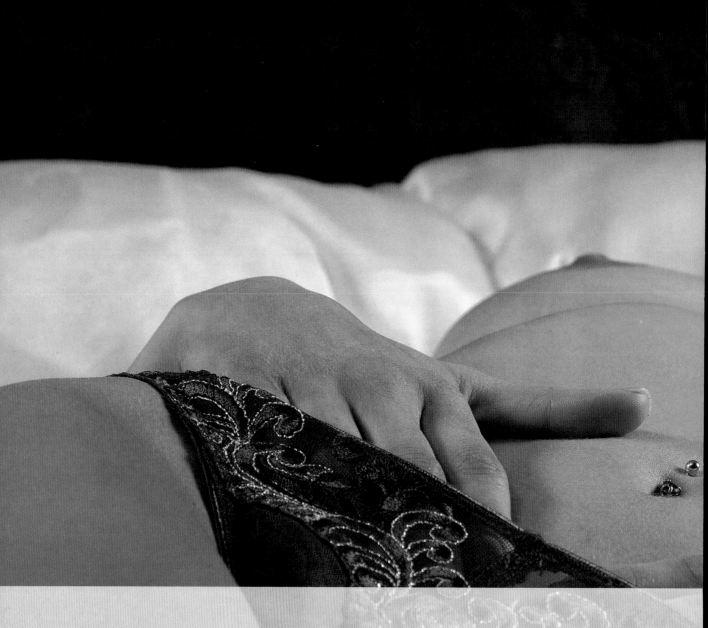

Chapter 3

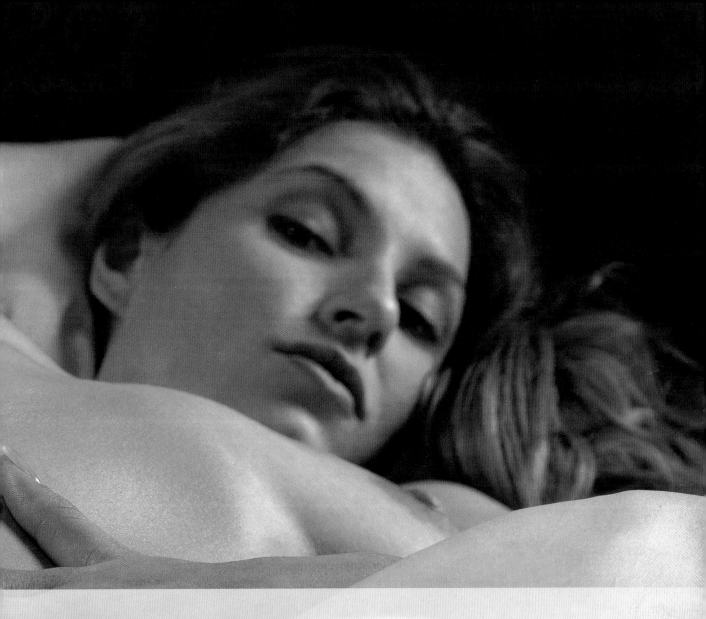

Her Private Time
and Hot Spots

Religious prohibitions aside, some women don't masturbate because they don't feel right about taking erotic matters into their own hands. That attitude is all wrapped up in the concept of waiting for the Prince to make them come. In generations past, women often didn't masturbate (except for the rare, furtive self-encounter) until their forties or fifties when, driven by either lack of a partner or one with erectile dysfunction and their subsequent racing hormones, they bought their first vibe. Now vibrators sell briskly to younger women as well as older ones.

Before starting this chapter, let's get a few myths and misinformation out of the way.

The following is *not* true:

- You can get hooked on vibrators.

- You won't be able to come any other way.

- If you masturbate, you won't want sex with your partner.

- He will be intimidated by your vibrators, so hide them!

- Masturbation is cheating on your partner.

- At the very least, masturbating means you are not excited by your partner.

An Orgasm a Day

I believe every woman should have an orgasm a day. Every woman! Every day! Single, married, satisfied, or dissatisfied. And she should own a wardrobe of vibrators—"sex life accessories," as we call them at Cherrybomb.

Why an orgasm a day? Because orgasm:

- Is a great stress-reliever. Like the progressive muscle relaxation technique, orgasm teaches stressed people to clench and release every muscle in their body.

- Relieves minor aches and pains, including headaches, by sending waves of endorphins—natural painkillers—throughout your body.

- Helps make you more comfortable with and knowledgeable about your body, which makes it more likely that you will orgasm with your partner.

- Relieves feelings of mild depression and boosts self-esteem (even if you come alone).

- Reduces the pressure on your partner to "give" you an orgasm during lovemaking.

- Makes you more, not less, interested in lovemaking if you have a partner.

- Keeps you in the game if you don't have a partner.

- Sustains the sexual response system for women over fifty.

Work vibrators into your sexual routine. They're a playful way to reach orgasm everyday, whether you use them solo or with your partner.

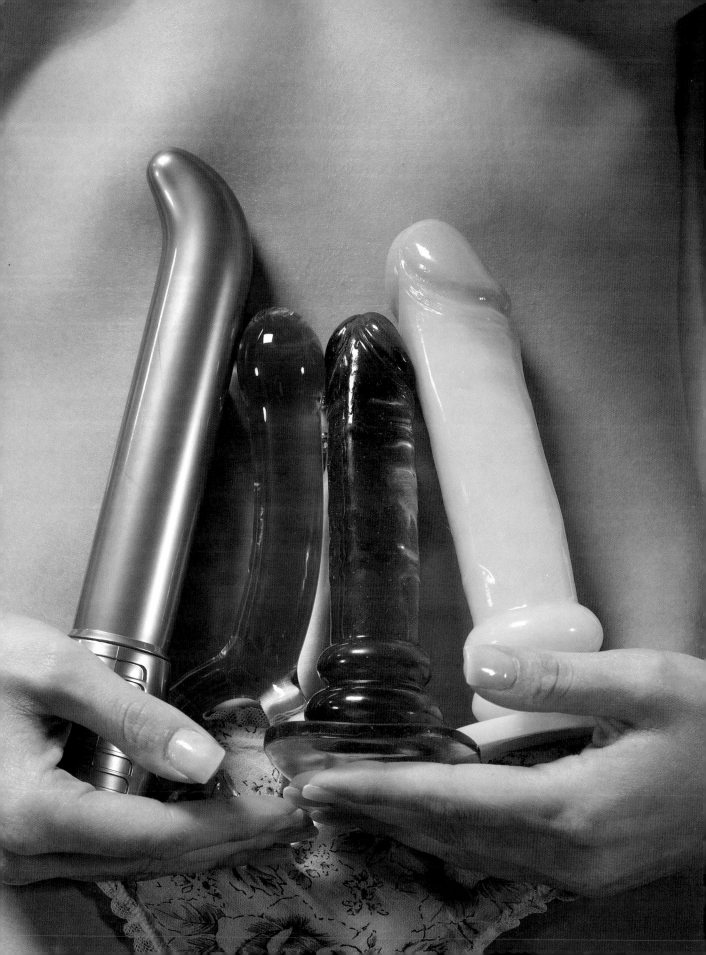

Finding the Hot Spots

Hot spots are those "magic button" places on your body. You have them. He has them. You know where most of your—and his—hot spots are, but you may not be hitting them (or connecting them with his) in the most effective way possible. If the hot spots connections are good during foreplay and intercourse, orgasm is more likely to happen and be more intense.

Explore your hot spots and discover how they react to varying stimuli during masturbation, and then take that knowledge into lovemaking.

The C-Spot

Nearly all women know that their clitoris (or C-spot) is that little pink glans (or head) inside the hood at the top of the vagina where the labia (vaginal lips) come together. It is sometimes compared to the penis because of its shaft-like shape. For the majority of women, the clitoris and the surrounding tissue is the most sexually sensitive part of the body. The nerve endings of the clitoris actually run deeper into the genitals than you might guess —making this the hottest of hot spots.

The G-Spot

The G-spot is that spongy mass of rough tissue located in the front wall of the vagina halfway between the pubic bone and the cervix and below the opening of the urethra. (Because you feel it through the vagina, the G-spot has been erroneously defined as being inside it.) It was named after the German physician Ernst Grafenberg, who "discovered" it in the 1940s, though this place was familiar territory to the Indian author of the Kama Sutra five thousand years earlier.

Can't find it? Place your hand, palm down, at the entrance of your vagina. Insert two fingers and make the "come hither" gesture. Nothing? Try squatting. Some women find it easier to locate their G-spot in that position.

Nothing yet? Try using a vibrator, either a special G-spot vibe or an attachment to one you have. That is the simplest and best way to discover the G-spot.

"I used to think that masturbation wasn't sex because it only involved me. That's a very limited view of human sexuality—and it doesn't work for women."

—Betty Dodson, the "Grandmother of Masturbation"

The AFE Zone

Near the G-spot is the AFE zone, a small, sensitive patch of textured, but not rough, skin at the top of the vagina closer to the cervix. Stroking the AFE zone makes almost any woman lubricate immediately. Explore the front wall of your vagina with one finger. When you feel moisture forming beneath your finger, you've hit the AFE zone.

AFE zone stands for anterior fornix erotic zone. A sexologist in Kuala Lumpur, Malaysia, rediscovered this area and named it in 1994. But, again, the Kama Sutra got there first.

The U-Spot

We typically don't think of the urethra as a sexy place. But the tiny area of tissue above the opening of the urethra (and right below the clitoris) is a separate pleasure point. Many women stimulate their U-spots during masturbation without being aware that they are doing so. Men typically discover it by accident while looking for the clitoris.

If you've ever thought, "That's not the place, but wait a minute, it feels good," he's hit your U-spot with his finger or tongue. And it's a good place for him to shift his attention between orgasms if your clitoris is too sensitive to the touch for a few moments. Try that after your first orgasm while masturbating.

Individual Hot Spots

Some women have very sensitive breasts, particularly the nipples. Other potential hot spots include the inner thighs, behind the knees, the hollow of the throat, and the back of the neck. After an orgasm, run your fingers along these places and others, and see what makes you shiver.

His hot spots are discussed in Chapter 4, along with directions for connecting the spots.

TIP

— • —

Play her hot spots like a musical instrument. While you are licking her C-spot, also stroke her G. Then move your tongue back and forth between C and U. Now stroke from the G to the AFE and back. Hot Spot Sequencing will drive her wild!

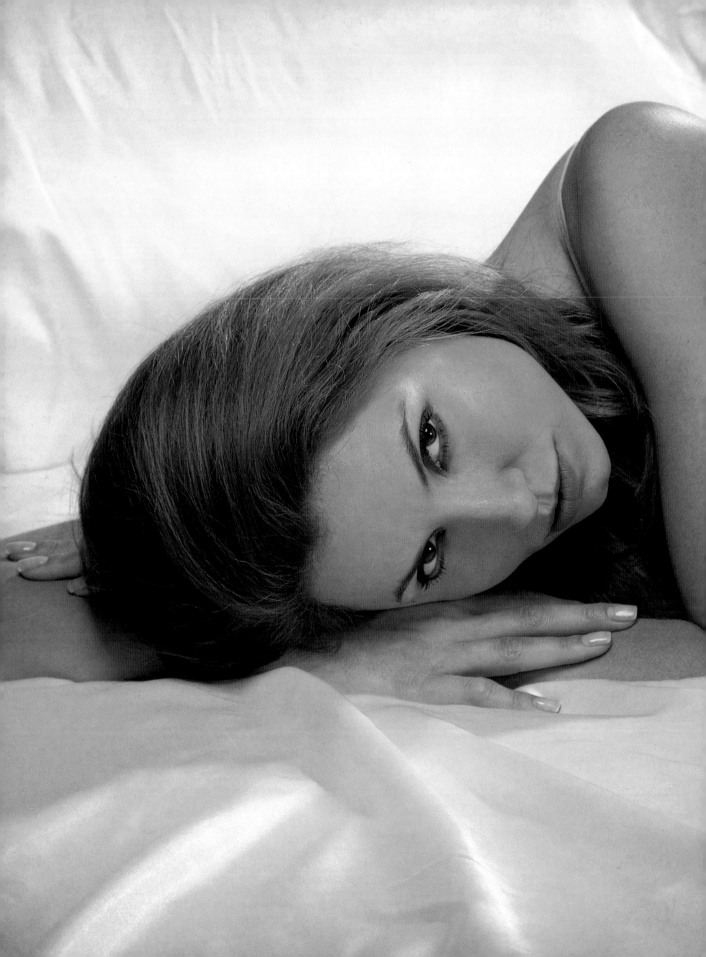

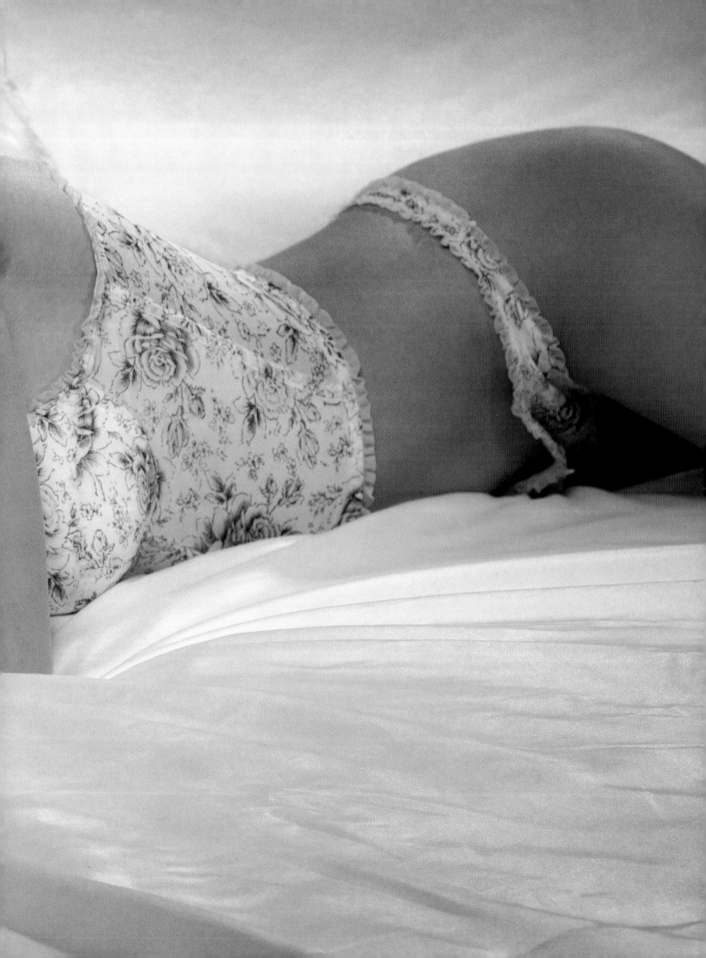

Why Vibrators?

Why do we like to play with vibrators? They're fun! It's all about pleasure—and pleasure is a good thing, not only for selfish reasons. You're undoubtedly a nicer person when you're sexually satisfied. If you need an excuse, I just gave you a good one.

Most vibrators are designed to stimulate the clitoris and are used externally. Some go inside, like dildos. Standard models get the job done, and quickly if you like. This is the vibe to use when you just need that O and don't have time for sensual or fantasy play. But you can also play as long as you want with them. Other models have more features.

If you are new to vibrators, here's a breakdown, including brand names of some of the best toys.

Hitachi Magic Wand

Often called "the Cadillac of vibrators," Hitachi is the largest selling vibrator worldwide. It's also a large vibrator. Marketed as "a muscle massager," it's available in drugstores as well as sex toy shops. And, wow!, does it make those muscles vibrate.

Eroscillator 2

The only sex toy endorsed by the legendary Dr. Ruth Westheimer, the Eroscillator resembles an electric toothbrush in size and shape. It oscillates rather than vibrates, so the motion is gentler against the clitoris, but still effective.

REAL TALK

How do you masturbate?

"The first time I masturbated I was fourteen. I'd been playing with the handheld shower nozzle, running water against my clit, though I didn't know what my clit was at the time. I got out of the shower and suddenly found myself straddling a bath towel, rubbing it between my legs. That's how I had my first orgasm. And I'm embarrassed to say that I still like doing it with towels."

—Kim, 44

———•———

"I start with my fingers and then move to a vibe. I like the feel of slick skin beneath my fingertips when I'm playing, but when I'm ready to get serious about orgasm, I like a vibe."

—Joan, 56

———•———

"I rub myself through my panties. The silk is delicious when it gets wet."

—Audrey, 22

———•———

"Well, sometimes I turn it into a big production, candles and music and the whole bit. But mostly I just grab one of my vibes and do it."

—Lisa, 29

"Hey, don't knock masturbation. It's sex with someone I love."

—Alvy Singer (played by Woody Allen) in the classic film *Annie Hall*

Pocket Rocket

Tiny but powerful, this one stows in a small handbag and gets the job done anywhere, anytime. You can change the texture of the vibe and the feeling of the vibrations by adding a jelly sleeve. Water Dancer is the waterproof version; it's great for combining the morning shower with the morning orgasm.

Fukuoku 9000

The top-of-the-line finger vibe, Fukuoku is a great couple's toy. Finger vibes wrap around your finger or fit over it and are perfect for clitoral stimulation during intercourse. Finger Fun is a slightly larger, waterproof version.

The Butterfly

A strap-on vibrator, the Butterfly stimulates her clitoris during intercourse while giving him pleasurable sensations, too. The Sweetheart and many other vibes, some remote-controlled, work the same way.

G Swirl

Designed to hit the G-spot, this one and others like it are limited-use vibes. If G-spot orgasms are your thing, this is your toy. (You can also buy G-spot attachments for other vibes, including the Hitachi Magic Wand.)

The Rabbit!

(Exclamation point mine!) Ah, the Rabbit, with its multiple joys, is the choice when you have the time and inclination to indulge yourself. Insert the vibrating shaft so it hits your G-spot and let the ears of the rabbit riding the shaft tickle your clitoris, as a vibrating band of pearls around the base stimulates your vaginal opening. Some rabbits come without the pearls.

Laya Spot

One of the many new contour vibes, the Laya Spot is both chic and ergonomically correct. Designed to fit the curves of a woman's body, it is versatile and discreet.

Talking Head

This Rabbit talks! The early version comes with computer chips—"lovers" like the French man and the girl who say what you want to hear. The latest version has an MP3 download, and you can program it with anything. On the horizon: an alliance with Clone-a-Willy that will produce a Talking Head shaped just like your guy and speaking in his voice.

OhMiBod

This is a slim wand that connects to your iPod and automatically vibrates to the rhythym and intensity of the music.

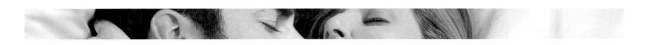

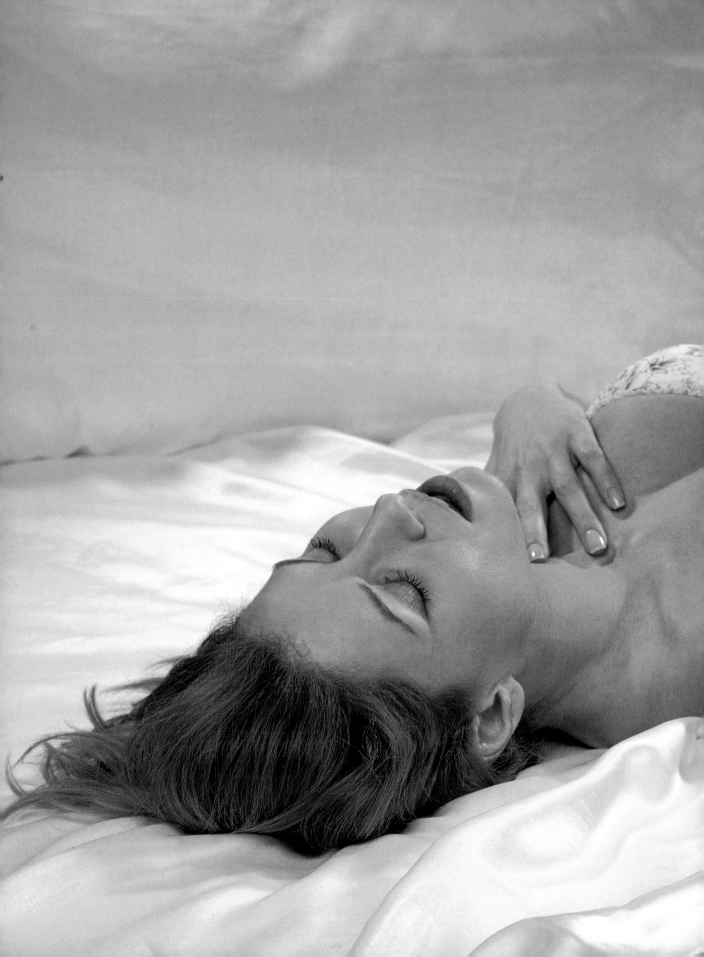

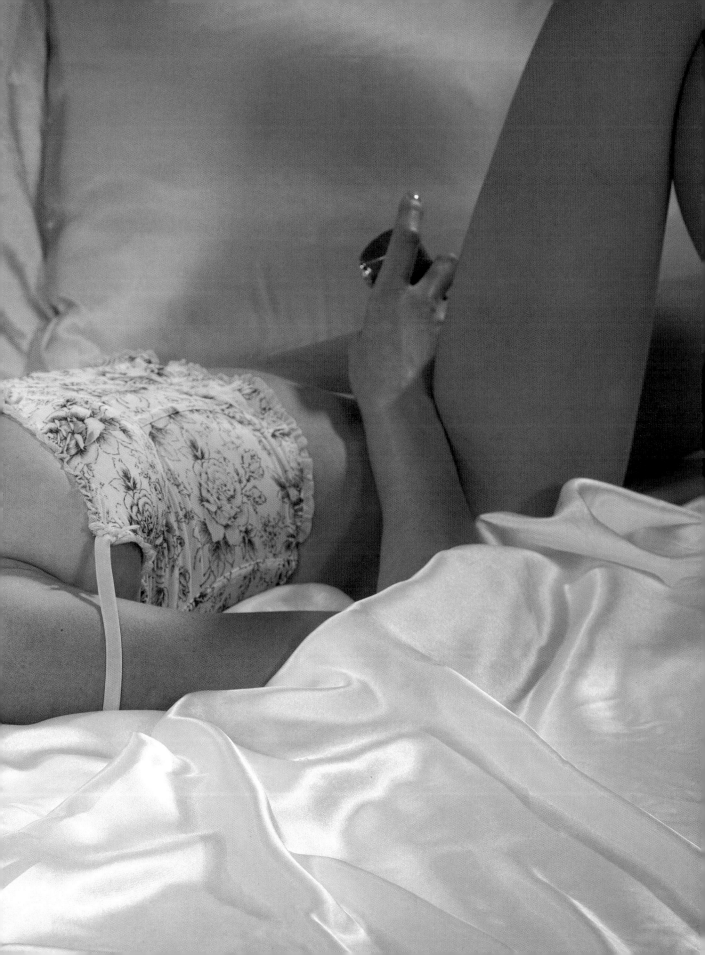

Mutual Masturbation

When couples masturbate together, they are usually in a playful, versus deeply passionate, mood. The drive to connect isn't so deep at the moment. What you want is a little fun and relaxation. Sharing masturbation feels intimate yet nondemanding. Watching your partner masturbate while you do can also be a hot experience.

How can you make it even better? Don't neglect the learning aspects of mutual masturbation. When will you have a better opportunity to figure out exactly how your partner comes?

If you are trying mutual masturbation for the first time, create a seduction scene exactly as you would do for "having sex." Dim the lights or light some candles. Arrange piles of pillows both for comfort and in good positions for the other's viewing pleasure. And don't strip naked if you're feeling a little shy. An open shirt worn alone or thigh-highs, heels, and a bustier are often sexier than nudity. Relax. Play some music. Flirt your way into it.

TIP

———— • ————

Add sex toys. This is a great opportunity to show him how you use your vibrator. Vary the types of vibes and the way you use them. And give him a toy too. He can wear a vibrating cock ring or hold a vibe against the back of his hand as he masturbates.

REAL TALK

"I asked my woman to masturbate for me. She said she would be too embarrassed. I kept asking. One day I said, 'Look, I'll go first.' She really got into what I was doing and started masturbating herself. It was one of our hottest experiences together."

—Carlos, 42

———— • ————

"I love to watch a woman work her pussy. You see the colors change and the moisture form. It's a sensual experience. And when I can do my thing and she likes watching me come—that's bomb."

—Andre, 39

Mutual masturbation is intensely erotic. Excitement builds for both partners as they pleasure their own bodies and get turned on watching their partner do the same.

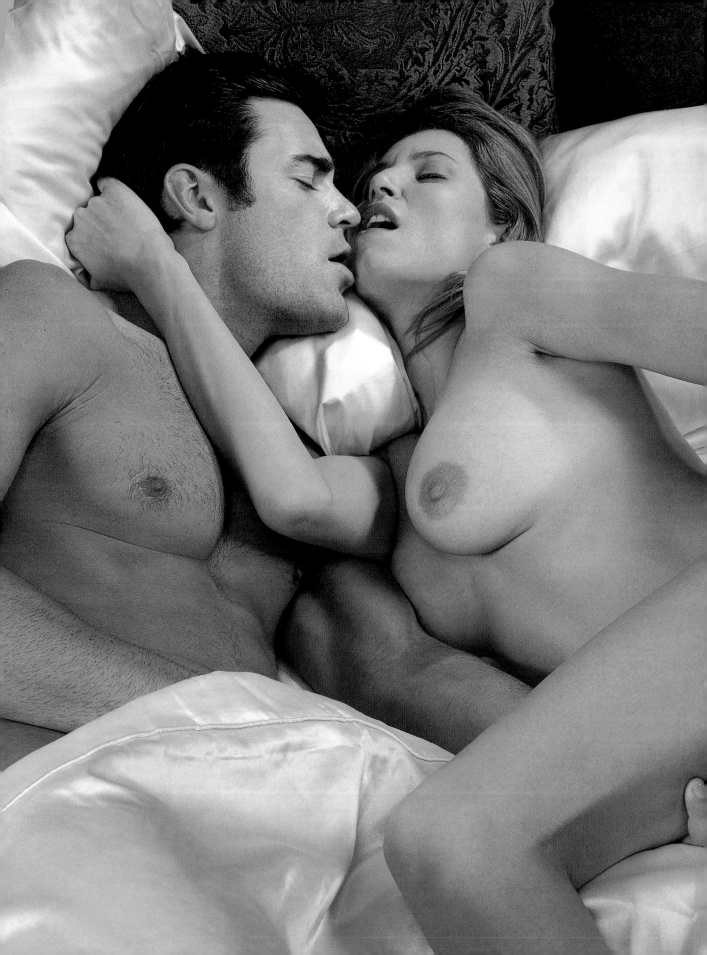

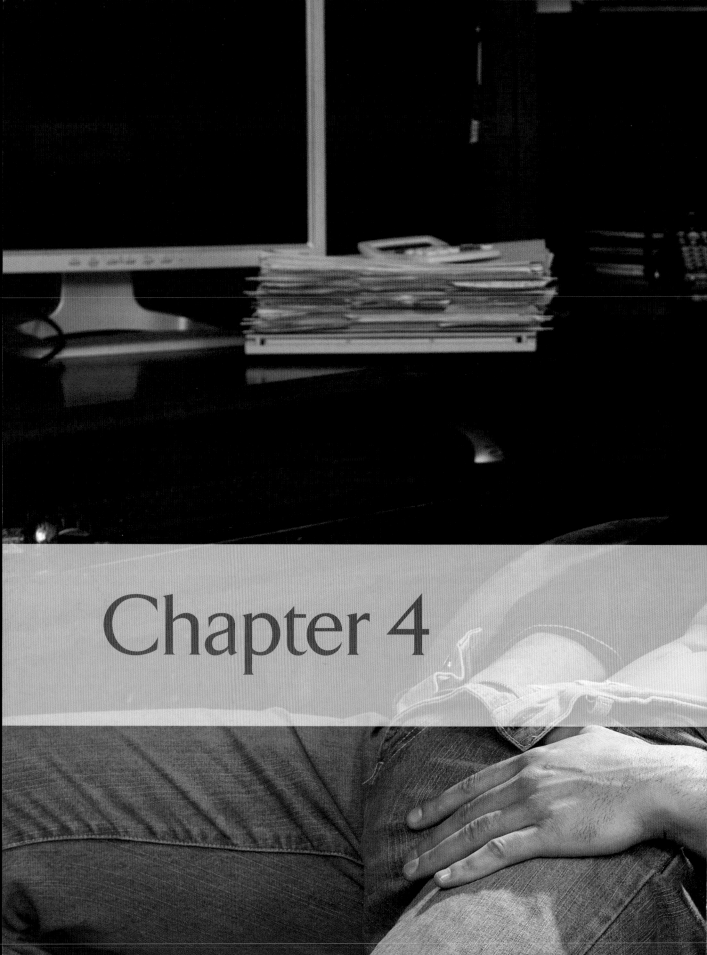

Chapter 4

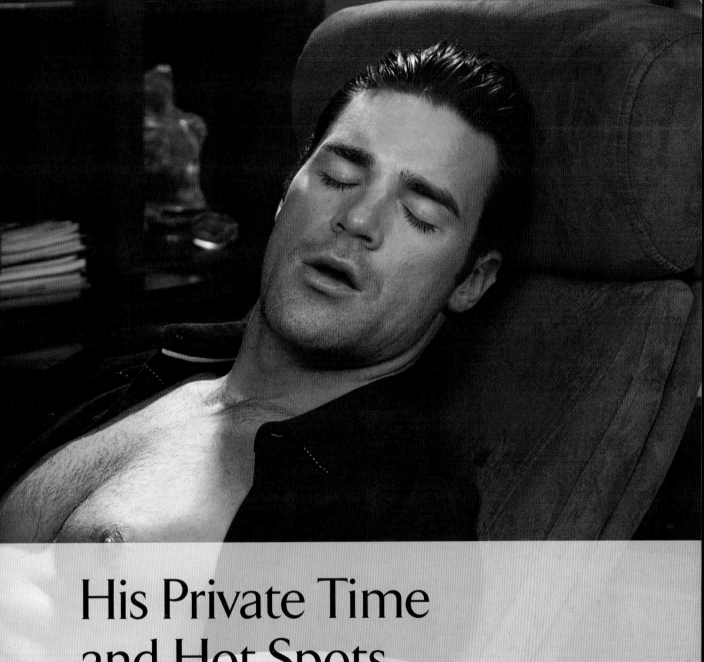

His Private Time
and Hot Spots

You don't have to tell most guys it's okay to masturbate. Unless they adhere to strict religious prohibitions, they aren't conflicted about giving self-pleasure, as many women still are.

Can He Masturbate Too Much?

You can do anything "too much" if that one activity is so obsessive that it prevents you from living a well-rounded life. But the odds are far greater that a man will be working rather than masturbating "too much." When he's in a monogamous relationship where his libido runs hotter than hers, masturbation is a good thing. If she's complaining that they don't have sex often enough and he's masturbating a lot, it might not be that he's a compulsive masturbator, but that something's wrong somewhere.

But what if he is masturbating in front of the computer screen while she sleeps alone in their bed: Is something wrong with the relationship? Not necessarily. Let's not be so quick to judge.

"I am going to my room to masturbate before a light lunch if you would like to come and watch."

—artist **Salvador Dalí** to a reporter who was interviewing him

REAL TALK

Why do you masturbate?

"Sex with my first wife took so long that I would sneak into the bathroom to masturbate rather than initiate sex with her. I saved sex for the weekends when I could afford to spend an hour getting her off. After we were divorced and I was with other women, I figured out the problem: A lot of women don't know how to have an orgasm. I learned how to give an orgasm after I was 35. My second wife is very responsive. She can come in a quickie. There are more options with her."

—**Steve, 49**

———•———

"I watch porn at the end of the day, jerk off, and go crawl into bed. Cyberporn and hookups—that's my 'love life.' I don't date. I don't have time for a relationship. Porn is ubiquitous, but it's the symptom, not the problem. There's no time to establish the kind of relationship with a woman that might lead to great sex. So there's porn on your computer."

—**Brad, 28**

———•———

"Masturbation saved my marriage. In my twenties, I wanted sex twice a day, morning and night, and more on the weekends if I could get it. My wife was good with four or five times a week."

—**John, 30**

Masturbation as a Learning Tool

We sex advisers are always telling women to masturbate so they will know how to reach orgasm. Men don't have a lot to learn about reaching orgasm—friction equals orgasm. Most of the time men masturbate quickly (and sometimes furtively). Take your time at it, and your sexual performance will improve.

Techniques for males to prolong masturbation—and later, sex—include the following:

Edge Play

Continuously stimulate your penis to the point of impending ejaculation. Then, stop. Yes, this takes some determination, but you can do it. Once your arousal level has subsided somewhat, stimulate continuously again to the point of impending ejaculation. Again, stop. Repeat as often as possible. Once you've learned how to prolong arousal during masturbation, you can transfer the skill to lovemaking.

Vary the Strokes

Most men masturbate in the same direct way, grasping the penis firmly and using a rapid up-and-down movement. That's why it's called "jerking off." Vary the strokes and the route is less direct. You gain more control over your orgasm. Try mixing in some of these strokes:

- **The Base Caress:** Slowly caress the base of your penis, squeezing the shaft and massaging the base.

- **The Slow Single Stroke:** Take your penis in one hand and stroke slowly up and down the shaft with your thumb or fingers from the other hand. Vary the pressure.

- **Circle Stroke:** Circle the head of your penis with the flat of your hand.

- **The Slow Two-Hand Stroke:** Use both hands on the shaft to perform the up-and-down stroke in slow motion.

- **The Cupped Hand:** Put the flat of one hand over the head of your penis. Use the fingers of the other hand to stroke the shaft. Vary the pressure and speed.

- **The Squeeze Stroke:** At the end of an up-down stroke, lightly squeeze the head of your penis.

- **The Open Hand Stroke:** Lay your penis in the palm of your hand and close your fingertips lightly around it. Use a slow, light stroke while keeping the hand open, fingers loosely curled around the penis. This feels more like a caress than a stroke, and slows you down. It's the male masturbation version of "take the time to smell the roses."

His Toy: A Cock Ring

A plain cock ring fits around the base of the penis and over the balls to sustain his erection. Made from leather or metal, it keeps the blood flow in the penis, restricting the blood flow out, and it can't be worn for too long. Vibrating cock rings are generally made of softer material. They also fit around the base of the penis and over the balls, but not so tightly. The attached battery pack creates vibration that is exciting for him, and for her, too, if he wears it during intercourse.

Trojan now makes condoms with vibrating cock rings attached. Other manufacturers produce disposable vibrating cock rings. They don't have the power of the bigger toys, but they are more than a novelty. Chic women now carry them in their handbags . . . just in case.

"We know that 80 percent of women masturbate and 90 percent of men do—and the rest lie."

—**Dr. Joycelyn Elders**, U.S. Surgeon General during the Clinton administration who publicly endorsed masturbation as a form of healthy sex

His Hot Spots

Like her, he has hot spots, those "magic button" places on his body. You know where most of them—both yours and hers—are. (Her hot spots are discussed in Chapter 3.) But you may discover a few surprises. Take your time masturbating and see how these places respond to different kinds of touch.

The H-Spot

The head of the penis is the man's big hot spot, just as the clitoris is hers. Who doesn't know that? Because the head is such a hot deal, the corona, the thick ridge separating the head from the shaft, is often ignored. But it is exquisitely sensitive to touch. Run your finger repeatedly around it. Doesn't that feel good? This is why the "silken swirl"—when she swirls her tongue around your corona during fellatio—feels so good.

That move, by the way, was a skill practiced by Italian courtesans in centuries past.

The F-Spot

The frenulum is that loose section of skin on the underside of the penis, where the head meets the shaft. In most men it is highly sensitive to touch. Some men reach orgasm more quickly if a woman strums the frenulum during fellatio. If this area feels particularly sensitive to you, ask your lover to do that.

The R-Area

The raphe is the visible line along the center of the scrotum, an area of the male anatomy too often overlooked during lovemaking. The skin of the scrotum is very sensitive, similar to a woman's labia. Gently run your fingertips along the raphe and see what that does for you.

The P-Zone

The perineum is an area an inch or so in size between the anus and the base of the scrotum, and it is even more neglected than the raphe. Rich in nerve endings, the perineum is the second-most important hot spot for some men. Use your thumb or finger pad to stimulate it. Start gently and exert a little more pressure if you like it.

The G-Spot

Yes, men have one, too. It's located inside the body behind the perineum. (I sense some of you getting nervous.) You can reach the G-spot in two ways: by pressing the perineum with your thumb or finger or by inserting a finger inside your anus and making that same come-hither gesture you would use to find her G-spot.

Many men love G-spot stimulation. Some hate it. You'll know where you stand by trying to find it first on your own.

Individual Hot Spots

Like women, you have your own individual hot spots, places of great sensitivity that lie outside the genitals. They include the ears, neck, inner thighs, temples, eyelids, nipples, and buttocks. After ejaculation, run your fingers along these places and note sensitivity. If you shiver, tell her where.

"Hot spots are personal pleasure triggers. Pull them."

—**Dr. Ava Cadell,** sexologist and author

Connecting
the Spots

You can make sex better by hitting each other's hot spots during oral and manual stimulation and intercourse. Why not devote a lovemaking session to mutual hot spot exploration?

Here are some suggestions:

- During manual foreplay, he can stroke her AFE zone, then the G-spot, and back again. Use clockwise, followed by counterclockwise, strokes.

- Don't overlook her U-spot during cunnilingus. Shift from the C-spot to the U-spot when she is close to orgasm. Tease her by going back and forth until she can't take it anymore.

- Don't feel badly that you can't deep throat his penis without gagging. Concentrate your attention during fellatio on the H-spot and R-area, while not neglecting his P-zone. He won't notice or care that you don't take the entire shaft into your mouth.

Make whatever adjustments you need to make during intercourse to ensure that you hit hot spot connections between her clitoris, AFE, and G-spot and his H-spot, F-spot, and R-area.

Here are some suggestions (the last two may require a little practice):

- In the missionary position, put her feet on his shoulders or pull her knees up to her chest and place her feet flat against his chest. Or have him hold her legs with his forearms under the knees.

- In the female superior position, she should either lean back or forward, which is more effective at hitting the hot spots than riding straight up and down.

- When using the spoon position, she lies on her side with her back to him, bent slightly at the knees and waist. Also bent slightly at the knees and waist, he enters her from behind.

- Try the X Position, which is adapted from the Kama Sutra position called "Woman Acting the Part of Man." Imagine that your bodies form an X, with the connection at the genitals. He sits at the edge of the bed with his back straight and one leg outstretched along the bed, the other outstretched toward the floor, or if he prefers, braced up on a straight-backed chair placed by the bed. She sits astride her partner with both legs braced on his shoulders.

- Try the Yabyum Position. See Chapter 13 for directions.

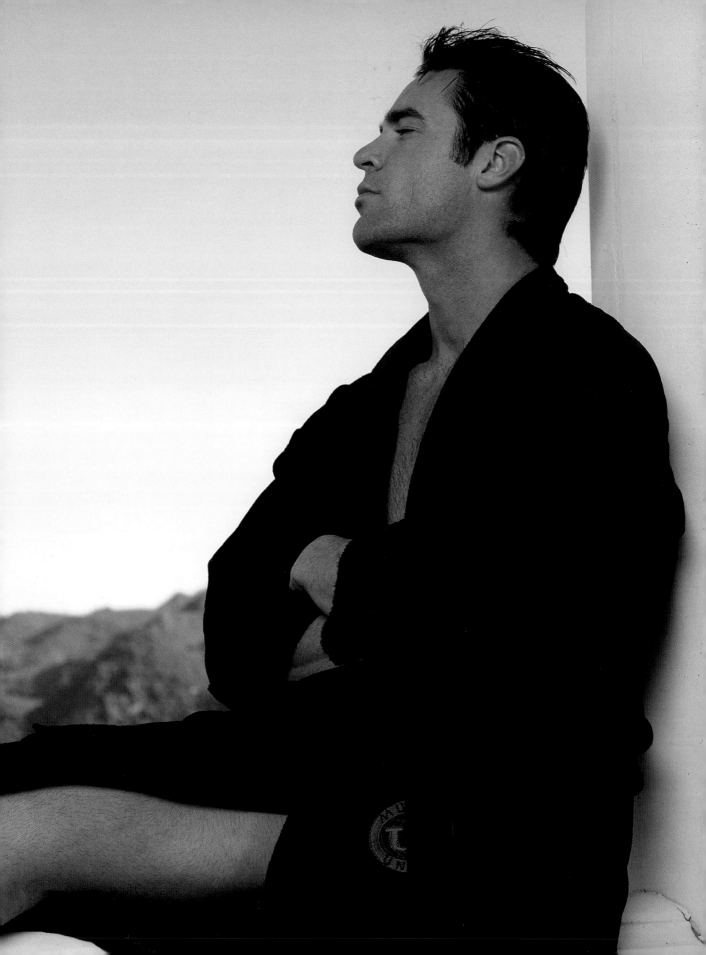

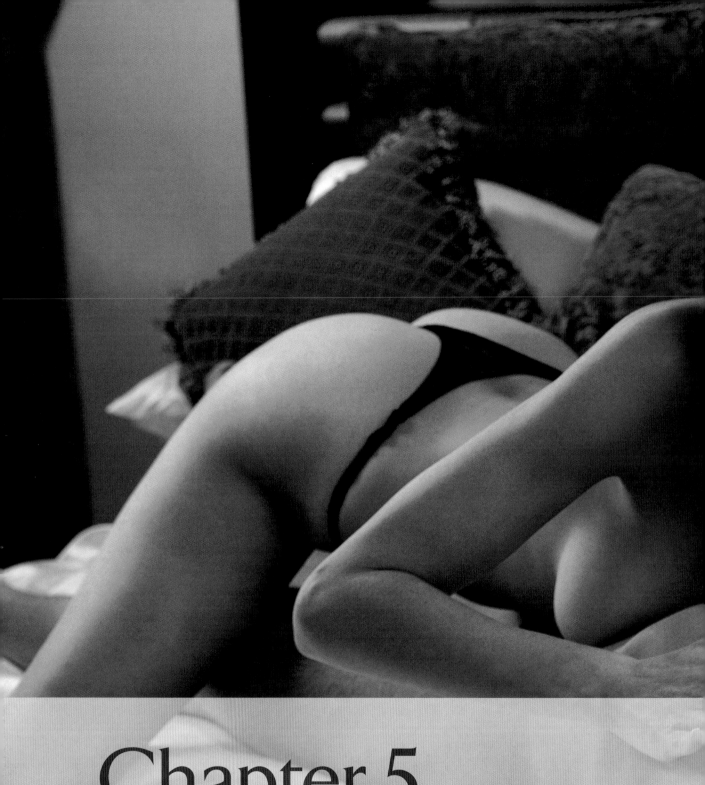

Chapter 5

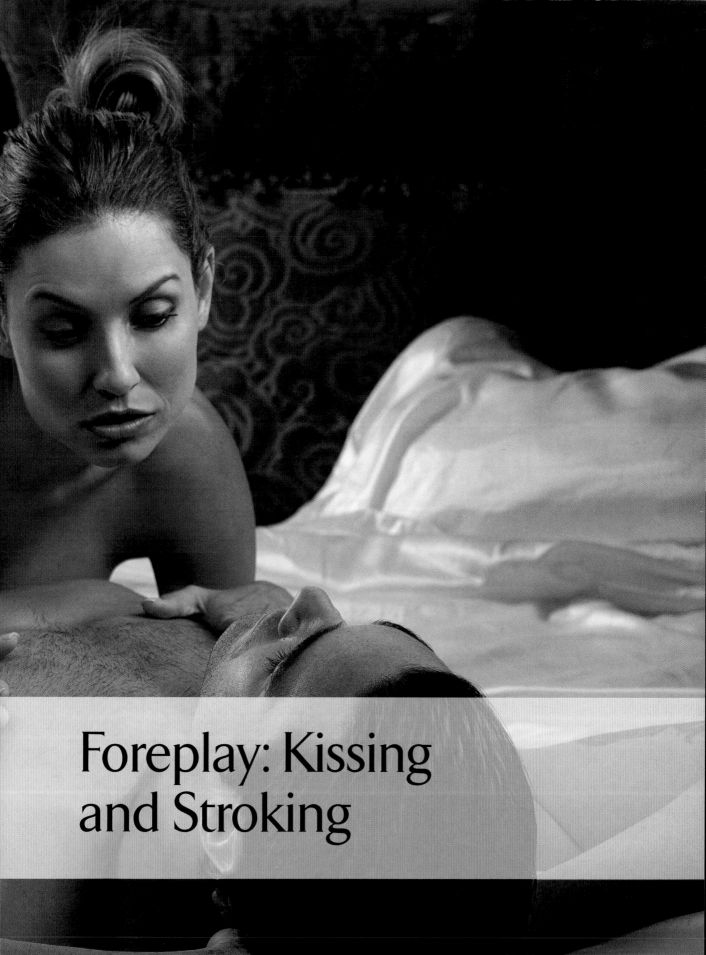

Foreplay: Kissing and Stroking

You must first seduce your lover's mind. Seduction, in fact, is largely a mind game. People who play it well know how to make us feel interesting and desirable. They know how to make eye contact—and when to drop the gaze. Look into those eyes and you see the promise of erotic fulfillment. Whether you just met the person or have been married to them for twenty years, their eyes convey something else along with passionate interest: a strong sense of their inviolate self. A truly seductive person is the man or woman you cannot own. He or she will share him- or herself with you, but not give it away. Now that is sexy.

Be sure to keep the following myths and misinformation about foreplay in mind (these are *not* true):

- Established couples don't need seduction.

- Men don't need foreplay.

- Women always need a lot of foreplay.

- A French kiss is full-on tongue.

- Kissing isn't that important after you've been together a while.

Foreplay: Orgasm's Great Prelude

Sometimes a quickie is just what you want, just what you need. You're both hot for one another because the foreplay has probably been going on in your minds for hours, maybe days. If she's savvy enough to masturbate a few minutes before the encounter, you will both likely reach orgasm.

Other times a little to a lot more foreplay is required. And on special occasions, seduction and foreplay are prolonged, turned into erotic events that could almost stand on their own if you didn't want that orgasm so badly.

Some elements of foreplay include:

- Building on the sexual tension created by holding, touching, and caressing

- Whispered endearments or naughty talk

- Kissing!

- Sensual body stroking

- Erotic massage (in longer periods of foreplay)

- Manual genital play

- Oral sex (which can also be an end in itself—see Chapter 6)

A high state of arousal usually leads to a more powerful orgasm, so take your foreplay out of the ordinary.

Eye contact is an important key to seduction. Look into your partner's eyes and see the promise of erotic fulfillment.

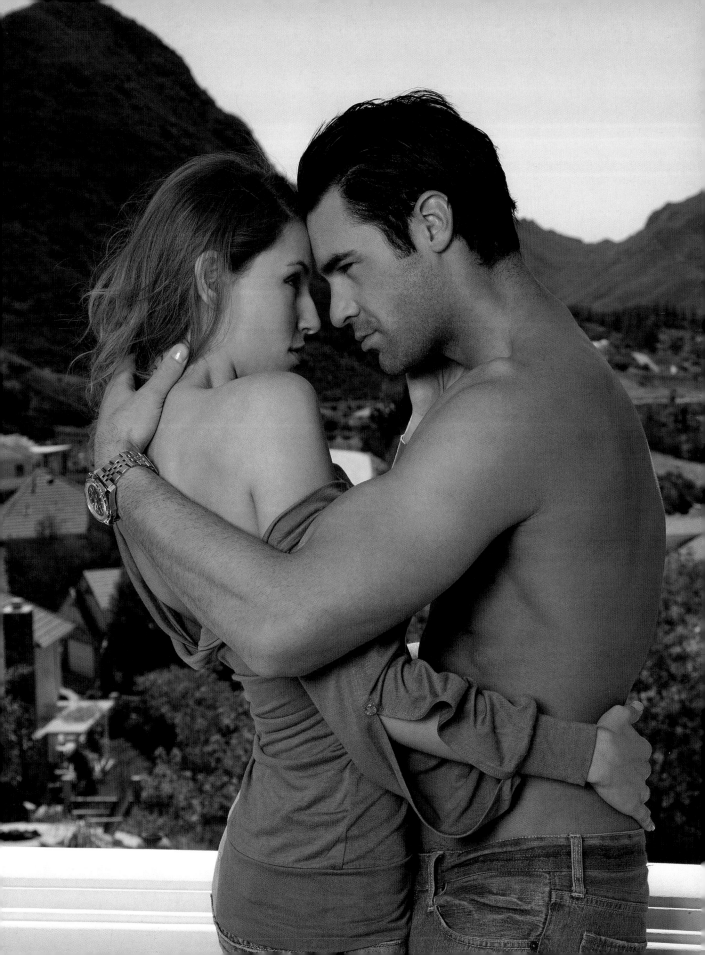

Teasing

Teasing is seductive. It can be visual or verbal. Teasing plays with the mind, triggering fantasies, making promises you may or may not keep.

The Visual Tease

From little things like unbuttoning the first few buttons (his or hers) of your shirt to expose the lacy tops of your thigh-high stockings when you cross your legs (generally her) to doing a slow strip for your lover, the visual tease is successful because both men and women are erotic visualizers.

Capitalize on that by "invitational dressing" when you go out. (If you look like Britney Spears in those panty-less Internet photos, you've invited too many people to the party.) Some things always work: her high heels, cleavage, and the glimpse of firm nipples beneath a silk shirt; his well-tailored suit, dress shirt open, tie cast aside for the evening. Some things work only for you. Figure out what they are.

Learn how to walk. He strides smoothly and purposefully. She has a loose, undulating walk straight from the pelvis. Here's how to get that—and tickle that Kundalini energy.

- **The Pelvic Bounce:** Lie on a bed or the floor on your back with your palms on either side of your buttocks, knees bent. Lift your pelvis slightly and let it down, bouncing your lower back gently as you inhale sharply.

- **The Pelvic Thrust:** Stand with your hands on your hips. Move your pelvic area in a circular motion to the right, then to the left. Exhale as you thrust your pelvis forward in motion. Inhale on the backward pull.

The Verbal Tease

Have you ever carried on an e-mail or text message correspondence with a potential hot date, only to have your fantasies smashed merely by the sound of his or her voice?

Voice is important. Pitch your voice lower. Listen to how you sound on tape. If you have a nasal whine or some other devastating accent issue, try fixing it.

Watch those sweet nothings and double entendres. They can sound shallow, foolish, or girlish/boyish. Verbal seduction is all about sounding desirable.

"What straight people call foreplay bears a remarkable resemblance to what lesbians call sex, and it's far more likely to result in female orgasm."

—**Ann Regentin**, writing on *Clean Sheets* online magazine

Try performing a visual tease—like a slow strip—to set the mood. Both men and women are erotic visualizers.

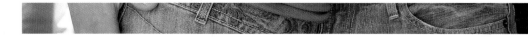

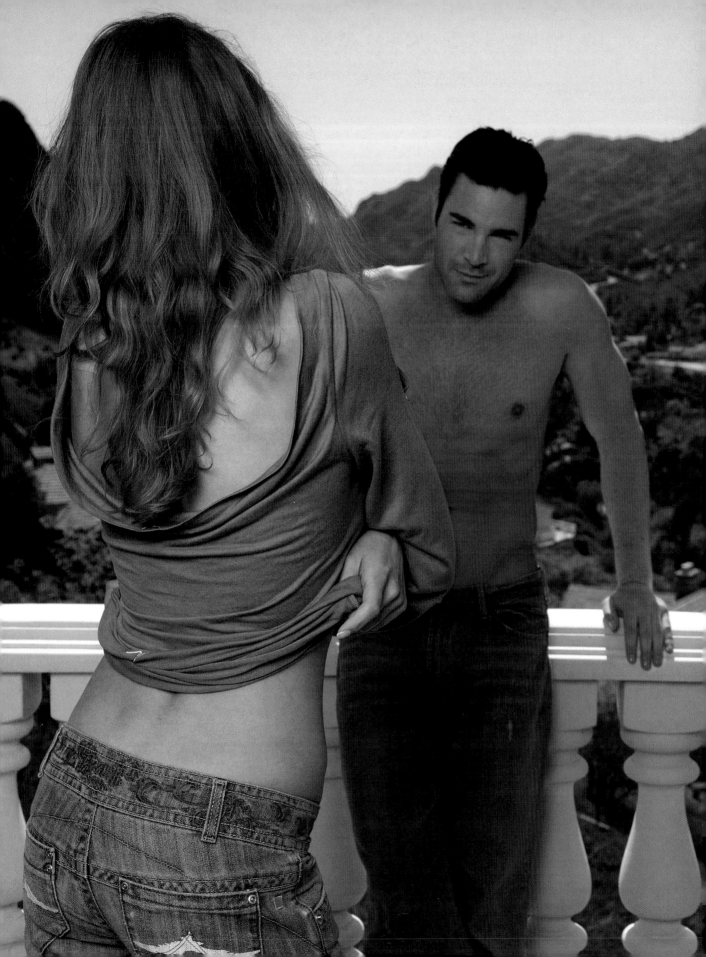

The Essential Kiss

If you don't like the way someone kisses or responds to your kisses, you're probably not going to find him or her an exceptional lover. The mouth is an erotic organ— visible, accessible, yet private. The kiss is important to men, but essential to women. Its power is so great that even scientists acknowledge the kiss is a form of personal chemistry, sending biological signals through the chemistry in our saliva. And too much saliva drowns a good kiss.

Start kissing somewhere else and work your way up to her mouth. Nuzzle her neck, lick her ears, kiss her throat.

If you are naked in bed, kiss the backs of her knees. Lick her nipples. Alternate the rough side of your tongue (top) with the smooth side (bottom) for different sensations. (All this works on men, too.)

Or if you are fully clothed, kiss the back of her hand. Turn it over. Kiss her palm. Then let your lips rest on her wrist until you feel her pulse beating in your lips.

Take her (or his) face in your hands. Brush your lips across hers lightly. Pull back. Put your lips on hers and press gently as you look into her eyes.

Explore one lip at a time with light, playful, teasing kisses. Gently suck each lip. Run the tip of your tongue around its edges, inside and out.

Now French kiss. With the tip of your tongue, play with her tongue, the inside of her lips, the edges of her teeth. Kiss her passionately, but don't assault her mouth with your tongue.

How important is a good kiss?

"A flabby kisser puts his lips on yours as if he were a piece of meat and you were a black eye. I can't get past a flabby kiss. If that's what a man's got, he can't get me."

—Claire, 40

———— • ————

"A good kisser is rare. Most men go in with the tongue right away—and too much of the tongue! But you can teach them how to kiss. I've taught every man I've been with how to kiss. I just take their face in my hands and say, 'Here's how I like it,' and I show them."

—Monica, 33

———— • ————

"The kiss is the deal maker or breaker. Men need to realize that. I take my time when I kiss a woman. She wants a sensual mouth experience, and I'm into that. But there is something women need to realize, too. If a man doesn't like to kiss you, he's not that into you. He just wants some pussy."

—Rob, 29

Remember that your partner's mouth is an erotic organ in itself. Kissing is important to men, but essential to women.

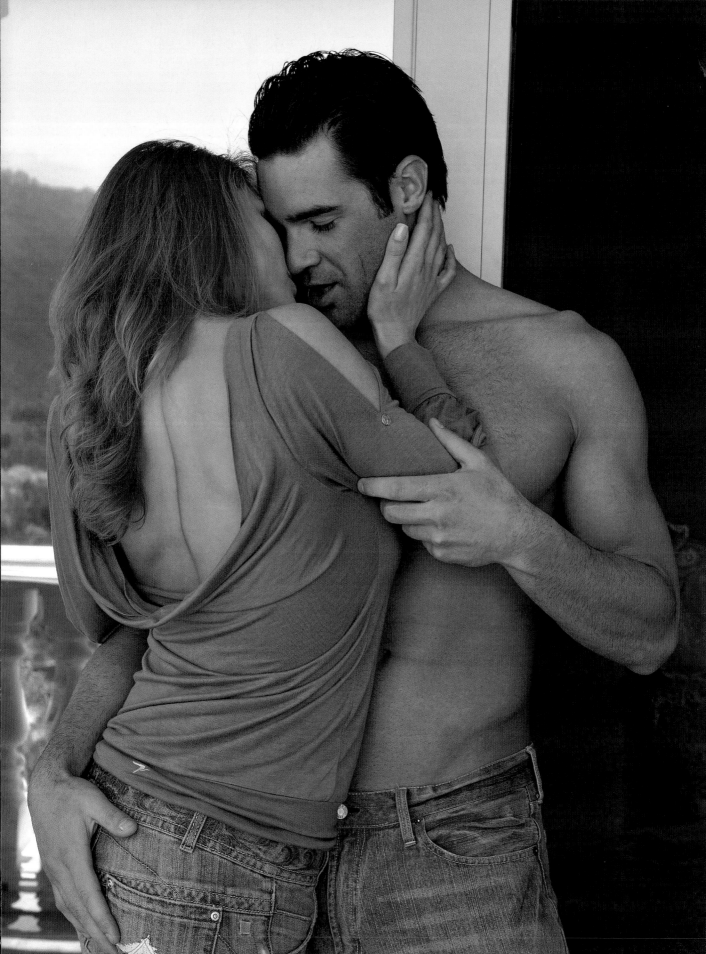

Touching and Stroking

What is the first physical connection you have with a lover? You touch one another's hands or arms during conversation. Maybe she straightens his tie. He brushes the hair back off her face. If the hands feel right on the other's flesh, the touches escalate. But if they don't, it all ends there.

Touch is a key element of lovemaking, yet few of us work on our hand skills once we get past the point of having our touch accepted by the new lover.

First, get the touch right. When you are holding your lover and caressing her (or him), touch her the way she likes to be touched. Most people respond to light caresses, with the pressure escalating as the excitement builds. Don't go straight for breasts or genitals. Stroke her collarbone. Rub his chest. Fondle thighs and buttocks. When you are naked, add some unexpected touches, such as the following:

- Using the pads of your fingers to play lightly over your lover's body

- "Scent kissing," or inhaling the scent of his or her body in places like the nape of the neck, breasts, and inner thighs

- Using feathers, silk, rose petals, or other materials to stroke or tease nipples and genitals

- Caressing his penis between your breasts

Hands-on Foreplay for Her

Don't go straight for a breast and squeeze hard. Pay attention to her cues. Does she moan in a good way when you play rough with her nipples? Or no?

Here are some strokes that work for most women:

- Before you do anything else, take her face in your hands, kiss her eyelids, and with one hand still holding her face, stroke her cheeks and forehead with your thumb.

- Massage her breasts with the flat of your hand.

- Glide your hand, with the first two fingers open in a V, up each of her breasts, catching her nipple in the V. Now kiss that nipple.

- Take her nipple gently between two fingers and pinch.

- Caress her inner thighs from her knees up. Let your thumb or fingers graze her vulva as you reach the top of her thighs.

- Don't forget to caress her back and shoulders, legs and belly, and all the parts of her.

- Use light circular motions with your fingertips on her genital area. Part her labia. Use your fingers to make long strokes on the outside lips. Then curve one or two fingers and use the space between the knuckle and joint to massage lightly her inner and outer lips in a back-and-forth motion. Massage her labia and work back to her anus.

Caress her inner thighs from her knees up. Let your thumb or fingers graze her vulva as you reach the top of her thighs.

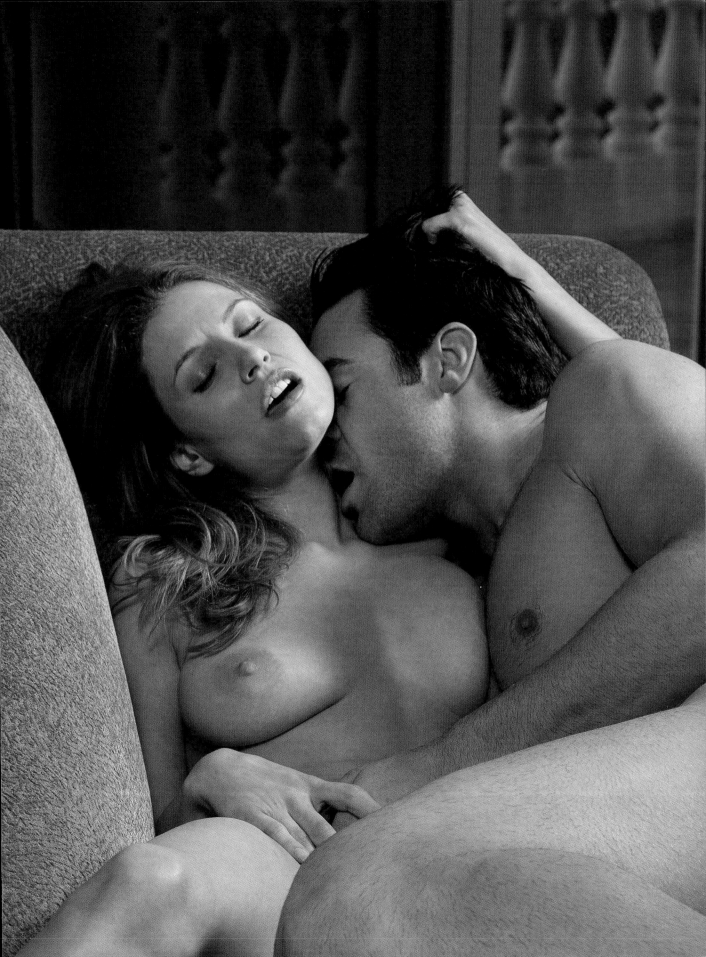

- Alternate that stroke with one using your thumb or first finger alone.

- Rotate your fingers around her clitoris, alternating a clockwise and counterclockwise motion. Stroke down with one finger on either side of her clitoris. Rotate. Stroke down.

- If she likes direct clitoral stimulation, you can take it between two fingers and gently rotate. But, if like many women, she can't stand the intensity of that stroke, circle your fingertips above the clitoris (at the twelve o'clock point).

- Add the G-spot stroke. While continuing the twelve o'clock rotation, insert a finger or two into her vagina and massage her G-spot (see page 44).

- Now circle your fingertip rapidly around her clitoris as you're massaging her G-spot. Don't be surprised if she ejaculates during this orgasm.

Hands-on Foreplay for Him

Some men don't like any kind of PDA (Public Display of Affection) whatsoever. Even in private, they may not be affectionate until they are ready to have sex. If he never holds your hand in the movies or puts your arm through his on the street or just holds you to be holding you, then he really doesn't deserve what you're about to give him.

But, like other, better men, he will respond to it.

- Knead his shoulders and back *gently*—not with the vigor of a masseuse.

- Make circular motions with your hands on his back, from the spine up and to the sides of his body. Alternate that with smooth, gliding strokes.

- Use single- or two-finger gliding strokes on his inner thighs, back, and the sides of his neck.

- Repeat the long, gliding strokes on his chest, stomach, and thighs.

- Do something entirely unexpected: Use the single-finger stroke on his face, even the delicate areas around his eyelids and ears. Also run your finger down his neck.

- Kneel between his legs. Take his testicles between your fingers and thumb them gently, one at a time. Then hold a testicle in the palm of your hand and tickle it lightly with the pads of your fingers. Now do the other one.

- Hold the base of his penis in one hand and work your other hand in a circular fashion (upwardly twisting, like following a winding staircase) to the head. Use the palm of that hand to caress the head of his penis.

- Take his penis in both hands. As if you were building a fire with his penis as the stick, use a rolling/rubbing motion, starting at the base. Roll/rub up to the head, keeping his penis between your palms. Use only upward motions. Start over at the base when you reach the head. Start slowly. Increase the speed as he gets closer to orgasm.

- Lean forward so that he ejaculates onto your breasts.

Use your hands to make circular motions on his back, moving from the spine up and to the sides of his body. Alternate that with smooth, gliding strokes.

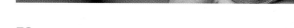

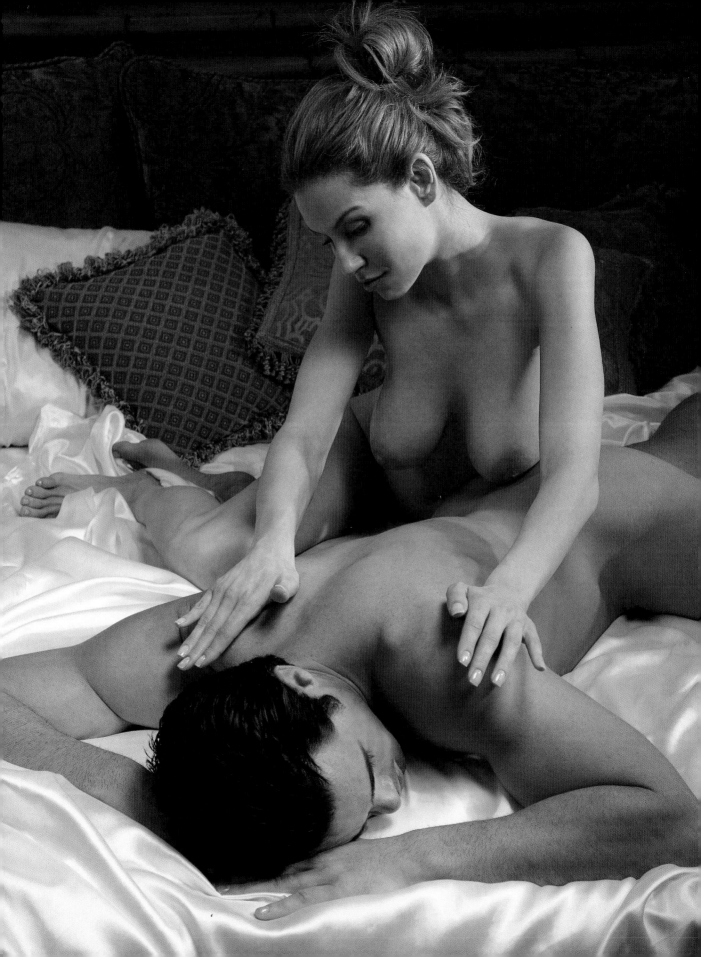

If He Loses His Erection

Sometimes he loses his erection during intercourse. There are four ways to handle this:

Turn His Attention to Her

He pays all the erotic attention to her. Kiss, caress, stroke, and fondle her—even bring her to orgasm. Go back to cunnilingus. Let your tongue take over for your penis. You'll probably have an erection after that.

Give Him the Stand-up Kiss

She performs fellatio or gives him a hand job. But even a good blow job or your best hand job may not be enough to wake him up on some nights. There is a move that usually works by combining the two, even if he thinks he's lost the will to go on. (The caveat: If he's drunk, there's nothing you can do to counteract those drinks hanging on the end of his penis.)

Here's how to perform the perfect "stand-up" kiss:

1. Hold his penis firmly in one hand. Take it into your mouth, moving the top third of the shaft in and out. Use the fingers of your other hand to stroke his perineum in a light, tickling fashion. If he responds to gentle scratching, do that instead.

2. When he becomes erect, use one hand to do a circular twisting motion up the shaft. Then start at the bottom again, as if you were following a winding staircase going up only.

3. At the same time you're twisting up, swirl your tongue around the corona (the ridge separating the head from the shaft). Alternate the swirl with the butterfly flick—flicking your tongue rapidly across the corona.

4. Continue the hand move while taking his testicles into your mouth, one at a time, and sucking lightly. Flick your tongue rapidly across his perineum.

5. Go back to the head of his penis and alternate swirling, flicking, and sucking. Remember: Don't take his penis too far into your mouth when you suck or you won't be able to pull off the suction.

The secrets to the success of this move are combining mouth and firm hand moves while not overlooking his testicles and especially his perineum.

Rubbing the Clitoris: Cowgirl in Charge

She grasps his penis and either holds it inside her or uses the head to stroke her clitoris. Combine a hand trick with the female superior position to create an instant, usable erection. No matter what position you were in when he lost that erection, get on top and give this a go.

First, straddle him. Grasp the base of his penis firmly in one hand, as if you were going to give him a hand job. Use the head of his penis to stroke your vulva and clitoris. When you are ready, lower yourself onto his penis without letting go of the base.

Grasp the first third of his penis with your strong PC muscle. Simulate thrusting with that muscle. (This alone may revive his erection.)

Lean forward, supporting yourself on one hand resting beside his body. (Your other hand still has his penis. Don't let go of it.) Work his penis up and down with your hand and PC muscle. Alternate that with what I call the "thrusting of the head" stroke: Use the head of his penis against your clitoris.

Whether he comes along for the ride or not, you will have an orgasm.

Try Heat and Ice

If all else fails, try a classic.

The late renowned erotic writer Marco Vassi once told me in the space of a commercial break on a talk radio show where we were improbably booked together that "running hot and cold" was a "mild form of kinky sex." Marco, who was beyond kinky and was on intimate terms with every bodily secretion, and I, whom he laughingly called the P.T.A. Mom of Sex, had almost no common ground except that we both liked to play with heat and ice. This is a technique that belongs in your erotic trick bag, too.

It's a great little pick-him-upper as well as just plain fun on a quiet night. And he can do it to you, too.

While performing fellatio (see Chapter 6), vary the temperature of your mouth. Start with normal body temperature. Then, using your hand to stimulate his penis, fill your mouth with ice cubes. Wait until your tongue is numb before spitting out the ice. Apply your frozen assets to his penis. This feels like a jolt of sexual electricity.

After a few minutes, when you oral temperature is back to normal, repeat the procedure, this time filling your mouth with a hot liquid.

This method of alternating temperatures restores erections in many men and prolongs arousal in some. Others say they have more intense orgasms after playing with heat and ice.

Marco's novels are largely out of print, but you should look for them anyway. They are awesome in their raw power.

REAL TALK

Have you ever experienced female ejaculation?

"The hottest sex experience of my life involved female ejaculation. I'd been trying to get this woman into bed for a while. Close, but not happening. Then one night she came over, we had some wine, we started fooling around on the couch. I don't know if I found her G-spot or what, but she came and she squirted. She said that only happened when she was really turned on and the guy hit all the buttons right. I've never seen it before or since. Man, that was hot."
—Dave, 48

—— • ——

"Yeah. I thought she peed on me. I'm still not sure she didn't."
—Chris, 37

—— • ——

"Sometimes I do ejaculate. It happens with a blended orgasm, G-spot and clitoral. It happens when I am so hot for the guy I feel like I'm going to explode. And it is not pee. You can smell and taste the difference in that juice shooting out of you and pure pee."
—Andrea, 29

—— • ——

"If a woman is a squirter, that's a problem for me. I don't like the squirter."
—Alex, 35

—— • ——

"I bought a video on how to female ejaculate —and my girlfriend hit me over the head with it. Literally. She won't even try."
—Nigel, 40

Female Ejaculation: Myths and Reality

Some devotees of female ejaculation—especially women who call themselves "erotic goddesses"—believe that every woman can learn how to ejaculate during orgasm.

That's a minority opinion.

And there are others, often men, who say, "Women—ejaculate?! I don't think so."

Female ejaculation isn't exactly a technique. Many Western sex experts dismiss the "ejaculate" as a myth—or a gush of fluid composed of urine and copious vaginal secretions. There is no question that whatever this fluid is that some women ejaculate, or squirt, upon orgasm, it is *not* the female equivalent of seminal fluid.

No, women do not ejaculate in the way that men do; however, something does happen for many women, though no one has answered definitively what. The ancients also pondered female ejaculation. Hippocrates set forth a "two semen" theory that, wrong as it was, has some basis in medical fact.

Men ejaculate sperm from the testicles via tubes that go through the prostate gland, where the sperm mixes with seminal fluid. Women, of course, do not have a prostate gland. But in some women there is a collection of several masses of tissue strung out along the urinary tract, referred to as the skeen gland. Medical researcher Josephine Lowndes Sevely wrote that in some women this gland produces a fluid that is neither urine nor vaginal secretions.

That seems to be the most likely explanation of female ejaculation, or squirting, to me.

TIP

If you want to try for female ejaculation, here are a few secrets. Intercourse positions most favorable for female ejaculation are rear entry and missionary with her legs in the air, his hands supporting her thighs as he thrusts. She should stimulate her clitoris as she angles her body to get the full G-spot effect. When the spot swells and feels more textured, she is ready. Hit the G-spot fast and hard. (If you're using hands rather than having intercourse, use an off/on stimulation pattern—again, fast and hard.) When she feels the desire to urinate, she should push hard instead of holding back.

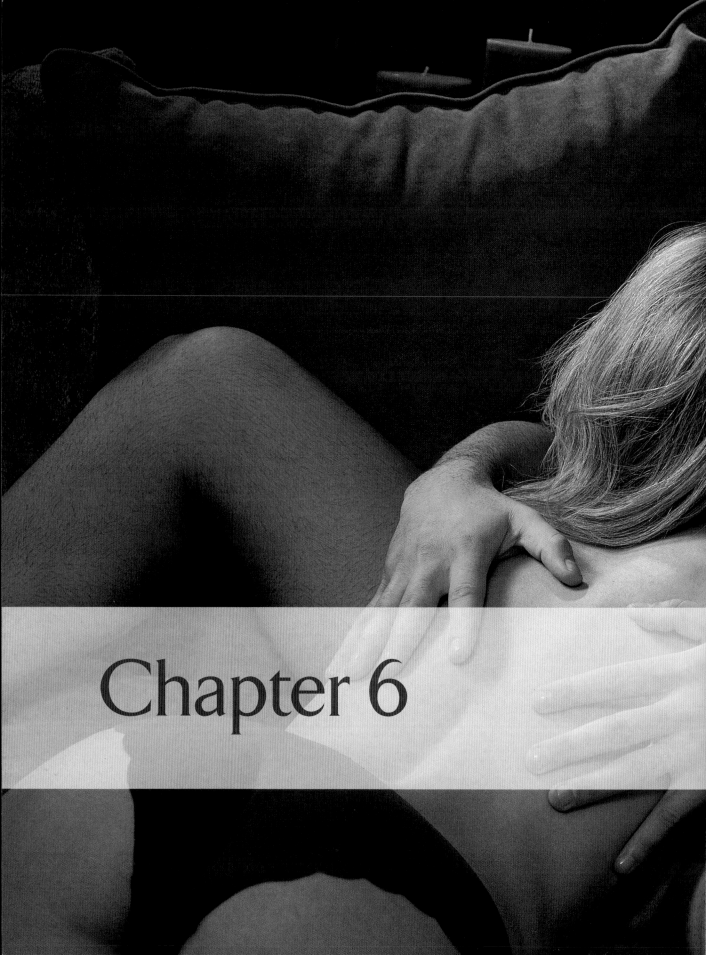

Chapter 6

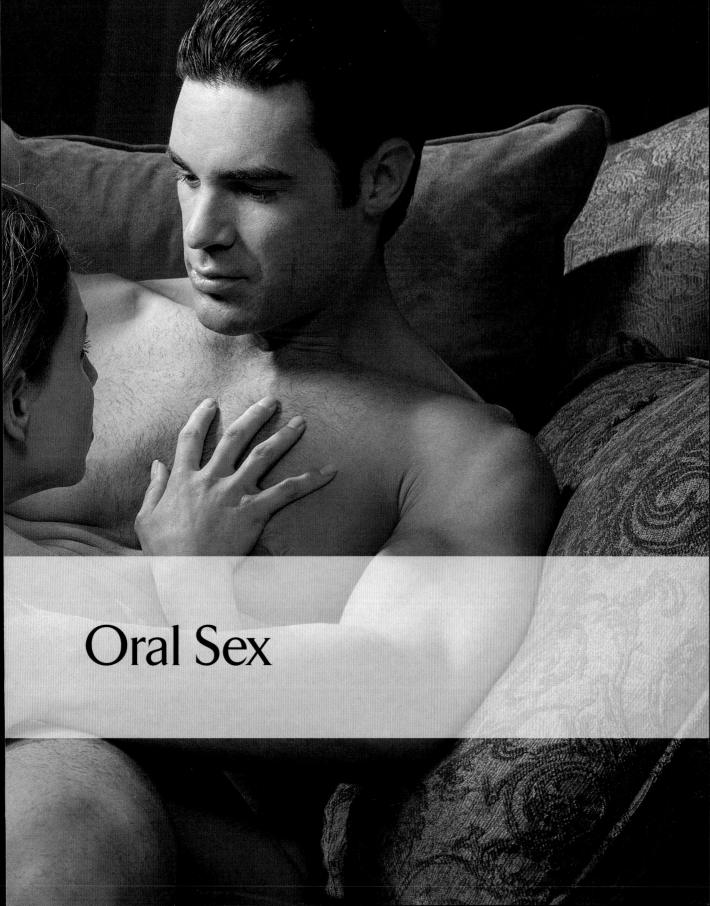

Oral Sex

Oral sex (like the hand job) is both foreplay and a sex act unto itself if you continue until your lover has an orgasm. Men often bring women to orgasm via cunnilingus before moving on to intercourse. Sometimes women opt to fellate a man to orgasm instead of intercourse. And fellatio is the fallback position when a man loses his erection. Given the popularity of oral sex, it's hard to believe that back in the 1940s and 50s, when Alfred Kinsey was conducting his groundbreaking research on sexual behavior, that only half of the men surveyed had ever had fellatio and far less woman had experienced the joys of cunnilingus.

You are lucky to be living in the twenty-first century, so perfect your orals.

Cunnilingus

Step #1: After you have kissed, stroked, and fondled the rest of her body to the point where she is very aroused, get into a position comfortable for both of you. She may lean against pillows either with her legs open, knees bent and feet flat, or with her legs outstretched and open, forming a V. You can lie or kneel between her legs or come in from the side and wrap her leg around your shoulders. Or she can straddle your face and lower her clitoris to your mouth.

Step #2: Gently part her labia. Holding her lips open, lift the clitoral hood. If her clitoris is well back inside the hood—an "innie"—gently run your fingers along the side of the hood to expose the clitoris. (You may have to keep one hand in this position.)

Step #3: Lick the delicate tissue along the sides and above and below her clitoris in long, broad, gentle strokes of the tongue.

Step #4: Experiment with your tongue strokes, paying close attention to her responses. She will let you know how much pressure she wants.

Step #5: Put your lips around the sides of her clitoris. Hold them in a pursed position as you gently suck. Alternate the sucking with licking of the surrounding tissues.

Step #6: If she likes direct stimulation of the clitoris —some women do, some don't—lick and suck it.

Step #7: Cover the clitoral shaft area with your mouth. Suck gently around the sides of her clitoris. Stimulate her labia with your hand or stroke her inner thighs, tease her nipples, or alternate manual stimulation.

Don't move your mouth from her clitoris now if she wants to reach orgasm.

After you have kissed, stroked, and fondled the rest of her body, get into a position comfortable for both of you.

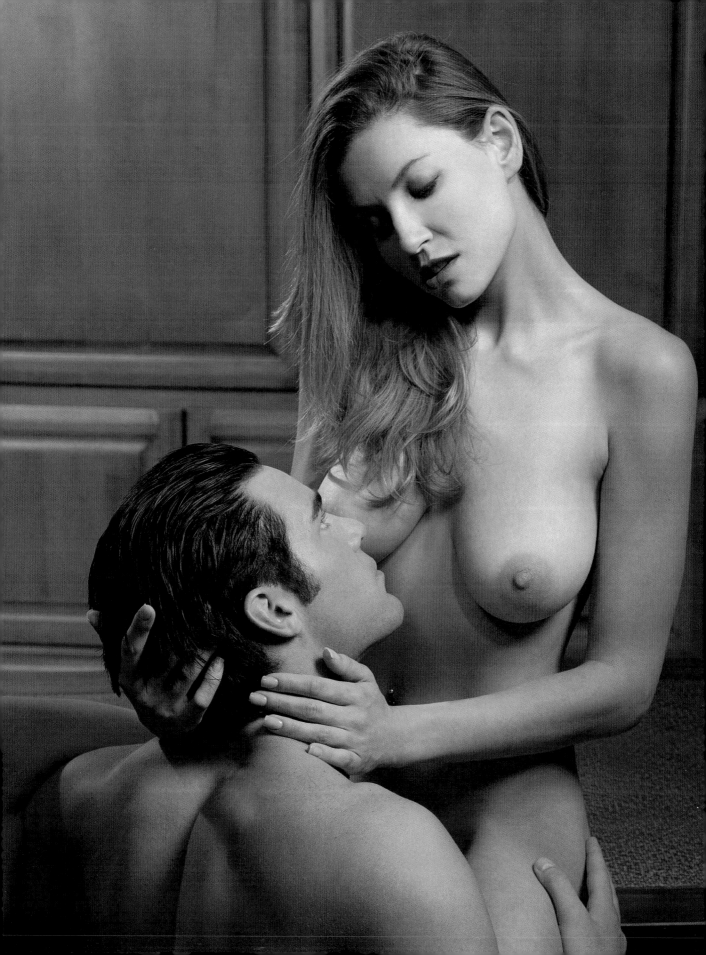

The Cunnilingus Power Move

If she's shy about cunnilingus, she may need to feel she's the one in control, not you. Giving her the power allows her to surrender on her own terms. Become her supplicant.

Kneel before her as she sits in a chair or on the side of the bed. Knead her buttocks softly as you bury your face in her vulva. Inhale deeply, and sigh happily. You are her willing oral servant now.

Begin licking from her knees up to her inner thighs. Manually stimulate her labia, vulva, vagina, and finally her clitoris while you give her thighs little sucking kisses. By the time your mouth surrounds her clitoris, she will have melted into you, inhibitions shed.

"I'll never forget the first time I ushered a woman into orgasm with my tongue. It was a watershed moment...both exhilarating and liberating."

—Ian Kerner, Ph.D., *She Comes First*

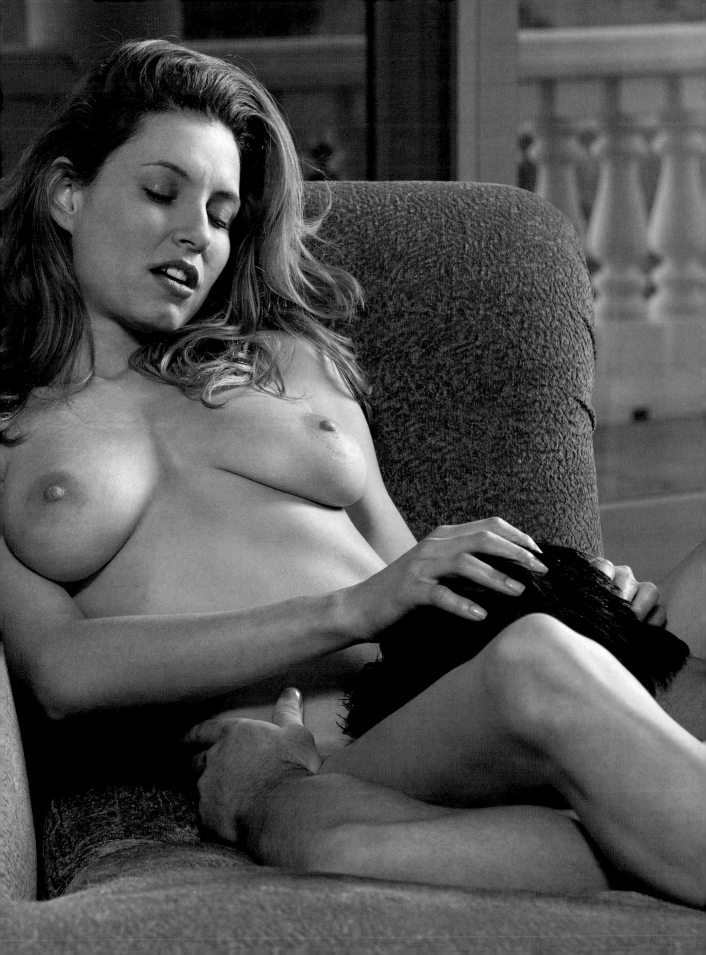

Giving a Great Blow Job

Step #1: Kiss and lick his inner thighs while pulling down ever so slightly on his scrotum. With your finger pads, scratch his testicles. Put his balls carefully into your mouth one at a time. Roll them around. Then, again, ever so gently, pull them down with your mouth.

Step #2: While you're attending to his balls, run you fingers lovingly up and down the shaft of his penis.

Step #3: Get into a comfortable position, kneeling at his side on the bed between his legs. Or, you can bring him down to the edge of the bed and kneel on the floor.Wet your lips and make sure that they cover your teeth. Run your tongue around the head of his penis to moisten it.

Step #4: Hold the base of his penis firmly in one hand. With the other hand, you can form a circle with your thumb and forefinger—what sex expert Lou Paget calls the "ring and the seal"—to elongate your mouth and prevent him from going in farther than you would like. Use that hand in a twisting motion as you fellate him. Or, if his erection is not firm, you can use both hands (wrapped around the shaft) in an upward twist stroke.

Step #5: Circle the head with your tongue in a swirling motion, and then work your tongue in long strokes up and down his shaft. Now, back to the head.

Step #6: Follow the ridge of the corona with your tongue while working the shaft with your hands, the penis sandwiched between them.

Step #7: Strum the frenulum with your tongue. Lick the raphe. (For more about these areas, see Chapter 4.)

Step #8: Make eye contact with him from time to time.

Step #9: Do at least 10 to 20 seconds of this showy move: Repeatedly pull his penis into your mouth, then push it out, using suction while keeping the tongue in motion.

Step #10: Go back to the head. Swirl your tongue around it. Suck the head. Swirl. Suck. Repeat. Repeat.

Step #11: Follow his lead if he pulls back from stimulation. He's telling you that he's going to reach orgasm if you don't stop.

Swallowing

If you don't stop, you have two options: Swallow or let his semen dribble out of your mouth.

Swallowing is not really difficult—and he will love you for it. A man feels totally accepted and loved by a woman who swallows his semen.

Position yourself so that his ejaculate will shoot straight down your throat. An easy way of doing this is to lie on your back with your head off the bed. Your mouth and throat will form a smooth line. Have him straddle your face for the elegant finish to the perfect blow job.

Does Size Make a Difference?

Oh, yes, it does to many women.

This is one place where even women who prefer a large penis can see some advantage in a small one. You can easily deep throat the small penis. Your gag reflex is less likely to kick in. And who doesn't feel like an oral genius when she pulls that off?

If your lover is well endowed, however, just concentrate on the top third of his penis. Supplement that with manual attention to the rest of the shaft, his testicles, and his perineum. Occasionally, adjust your position to allow you to take in all or most of his length.

Here are a few ways to do this:

- Kneel in front of him, bringing your mouth straight over the head of his penis. Now lower your head, taking in as much of him as you're comfortable with.

- Have him lie on his side. Now you lie beside him with your head at penis level and take him into your mouth. The sideways angle gives you more control because he doesn't thrust as vigorously into your mouth as he does when he's flat on his back.

- Lie on your back with your head over the edge of the bed. Have him kneel over you and thrust gently into your mouth. Control the depth of penetration with the ring and the seal.

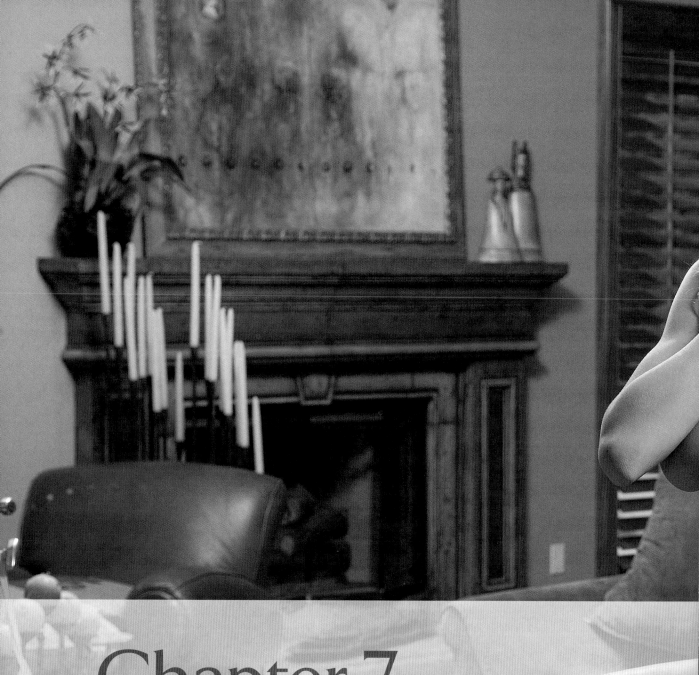

Chapter 7

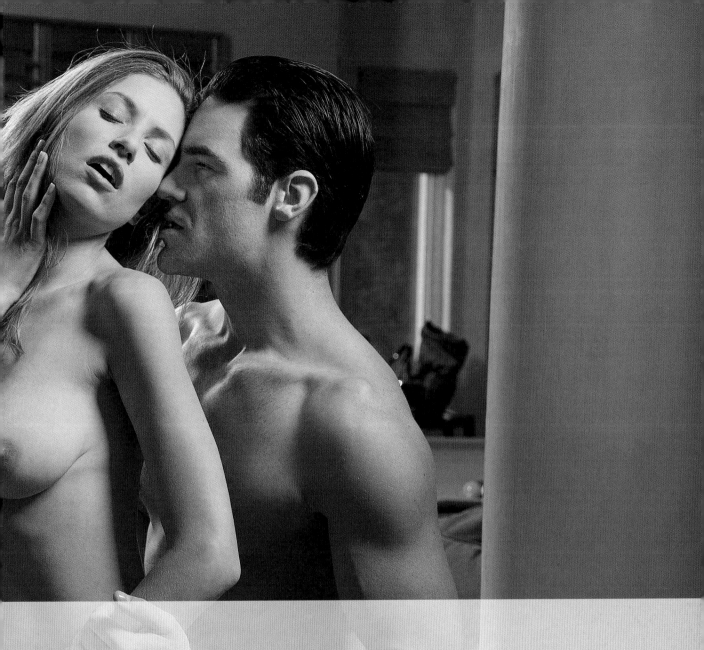

Games for Grown-ups

Foreplay is where you put the "play" back in sex. This chapter gives you some suggestions for doing that in a fun way through seduction games. Think how many ways you knew how to play when you were a kid. Games came naturally to you then—before you were serious about bills, chores, and relationships. Now you can learn how to play again.

Public Foreplay

You've seen that couple who can't keep their hands off each other in a restaurant, at a party, anywhere in public. Maybe you've been that couple. Pick a dark booth in your neighborhood bar. Kick off your shoe and play with his leg—all the way up his leg. Sit on his lap on a park bench and make out. Kiss and fondle one another on the beach at night.

A little public exposure will boost your libido.

TIP

———— • ————

Do what you did before sex became routine. Hold your hand on the small of her back and lightly press your finger pads against her. Rest your hand on his thigh with your thumb inside his leg and pointing toward his genitals. Nuzzle her neck. Put your hand flat on his chest as you're talking to him. Re-capture the feeling.

What kind of foreplay games do you play?

"I know this sounds really silly but we chase each other around the apartment. The one who wants sex chases; the one who is less into it runs away. All that running around gets the blood pumping. Plus, whoever gets caught has to take off an item of clothing."

—Ben, 23

———— • ————

"We tease each other a lot, especially when one of us is horny. We drop double entendres. Making dinner together, we bump into each other a lot. And we play 'grab ass,' which is something I remember my parents did when I was a little kid."

—Melanie, 34

———— • ————

"She's the one who is good at games. When she wants to seduce me, she dresses the part and struts like a catwalk model while keeping her face impassive."

—Kevin, 46

———— • ————

"Two words: Strip Monopoly."

—Cal, 29

Car Sex

Now what is more redolent of American youth than sex in a car?

You don't have to park on a lover's lane. The driveway or garage will do. There's nothing like the feel of a gearshift in your back—or the sight of her bare feet against the window.

Part of the thrill is in the limited range of motion. The car is a great place to give head, have sex in the sitting position, or wrap her legs around his neck. The space is tight—and that feels illicit.

Bump and Grind

Standing fully dressed, kiss and caress each other with your pelvises pressed together. When you feel the steam rising between the two of you, she bumps into him on the upstroke and grinds into him on the downstroke. Wrap one leg around his waist or use a door or wall for balance—but don't lie down.

Outercourse

Remember when you were a teenager and you made out on the family room floor while your parents were sleeping upstairs? You kept your clothes on—the better for a quick recovery if your parents came in. And it was really hot. Take it all the way to dry humping. It's thrilling to have an orgasm with your clothes on.

Striptease

Do you undress in the bathroom? Or with the lights off? Or just hurriedly get out of your clothes, barely looking at one another as you strip for sleep?

Put the drama back into undressing, especially if you're dressed up. Take off your skirt first and walk around in heels and stockings before taking off your blouse.

And remember tripping works both ways. Let her take in your bare chest and broad shoulders. When you step out of your pants, look her straight in the eye.

"Sex should be fun. It should be play. What it should not be is 'work.' The concept of working on the sex is very Puritan."

—**Trina Morgan, Ph.D.**, sex therapist and psychologist

The Office Call

If either of you has a private office—the sort where the door actually closes—or sometimes works late at night alone in the office, you have a perfect opportunity to play Office Call. The partner paying the call is responsible for the party. Maybe that includes refreshments, maybe not. But your picnic basket should contain treats like Honey Dust, a vibrating cock ring, a finger vibe, or whatever toys work quickly for you.

Clear off the desk, take off your coat, and enjoy.

TIP

— . —

Use the Master/Mistress and Slave game to explore hidden facets of your sexual personality. Role-playing allows you to play submissive or dominant in a relationship that is most likely based on erotic egalitarianism. But you must take turns being the dom and the sub. Keep it light. For example, tell your slave that she must submit to an erotic spanking or that he must kneel before you and give you oral pleasure until you orgasm. Script your roles. He can be the pirate ravishing the captured beauty. Or she can be the secret agent using her wiles to get an informant to talk.

Silly Sex Games that Work...

. . . but not always. If she feels silly doing them, they won't work. And if he feels like the little games are part of some grand entrapment plan, they won't work either. Do these only if you can carry them off in the spirit of fun.

- Send naughty text messages to one another.

- When you dress to leave, "forget" your panties or briefs.

- Apply an erotic temporary tattoo to your body—and make him or her find it.

- Eat off one another's naked bodies.

- Find sexy adult games online and play them.

- Play Strip Anything. (It doesn't have to be poker.)

- Assign some sex acts as "rewards" or "punishments" for losing at tennis, being late for a dinner date, or whatever.

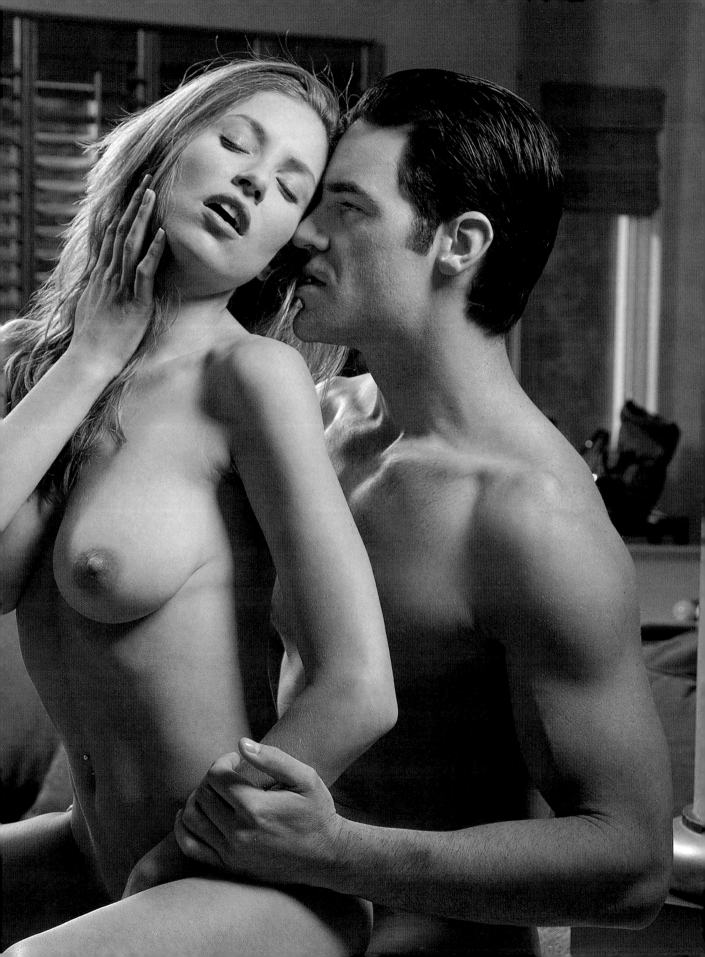

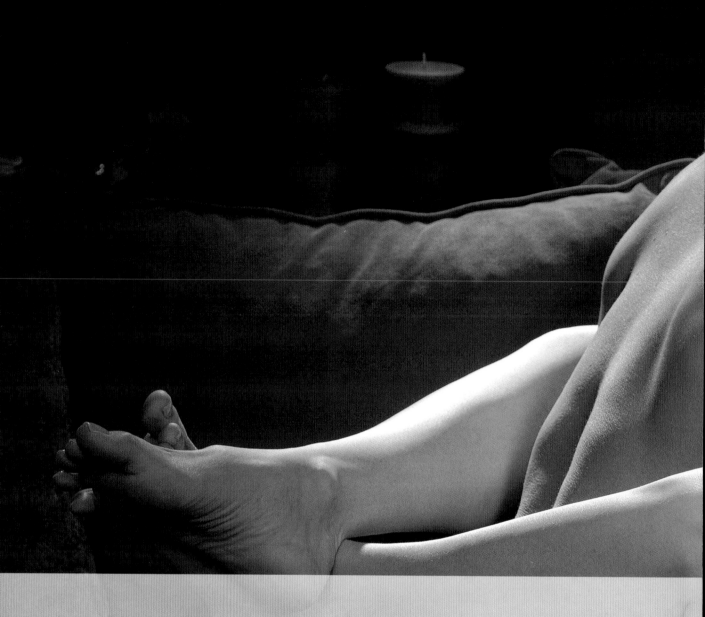

Chapter 8

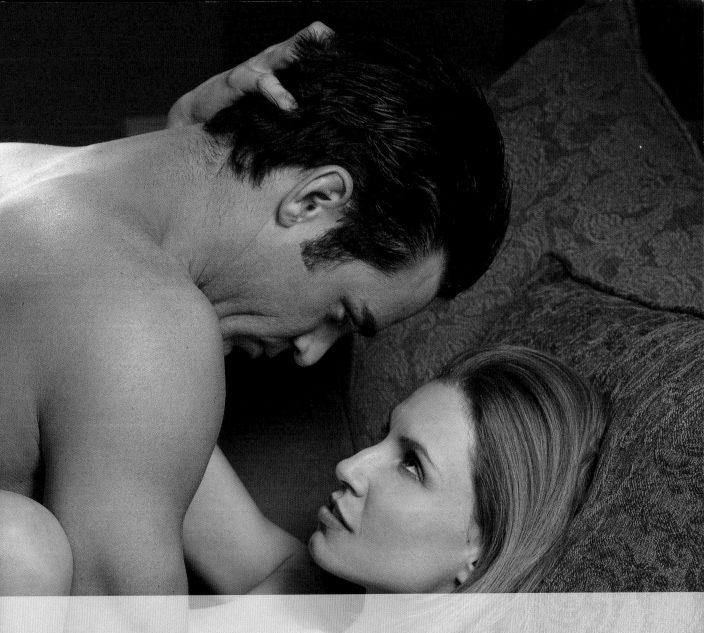

About Her Orgasms

And you are so ready to come now, aren't you? So ready that you are impatient for the instant gratification formula? If you have trouble reaching orgasm, you will learn how to get there more reliably and in less time by reading this chapter. If you want stronger, longer orgasms, you can get those, too, if you really want them.

But the one perfect "instant gratification," one-size-fits-all formula does continue to elude science and sex advisors. There are a lot of theories—many conflicting—about orgasm, mostly female orgasm. Partly that is because no one set of instructions on how to reach orgasm fits all women (or men) all the time, throughout their lives. Sexual response varies so much from one person or situation to another that no "answer" applies universally.

That said, you will find something here that does it for you. Try on theories and play around with techniques until you find the right combination for you. One thing I can say definitively: The female orgasm is not elusive. It's right beneath your fingertips.

"Orgasms are electrifying and mysterious. Why do orgasms feel so good? What inhibits them? Do men and women's orgasms differ? How many kinds are there? Does aging affect orgasm?"

—**Helen Fisher, Ph.D.,** *Why We Love*

TIP

Beyond the clitoris and the G-spot, the "new" orgasm trigger may be your cervix—the opening of your uterus. Studies have shown that up to half of women may reach orgasm through repeated thrusting against the cervix. The catch? Unless a man is exceptionally well endowed or the couple is in the right position, his penis isn't likely to touch her cervix during intercourse. The best position for cervical stimulation is this: She lies on her back with her legs drawn up. This shortens her vaginal canal—giving his penis a better chance of making contact.

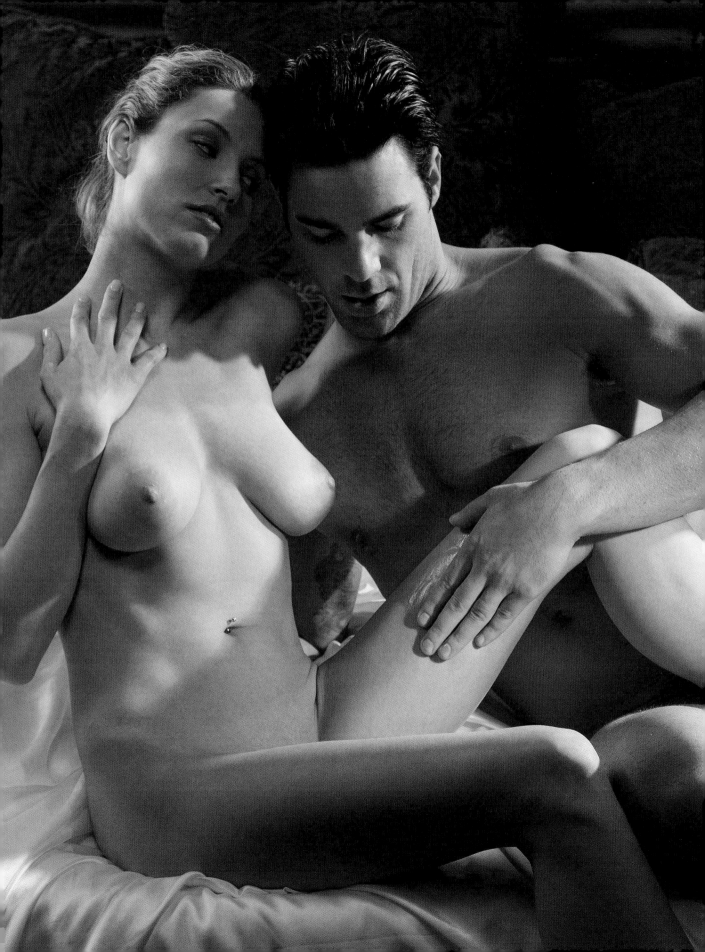

Why Orgasm?

Biologically speaking, the answer is simple for his orgasm: procreation. He has an orgasm and ejaculates, sending his sperm out to meet their fate.

But she doesn't need an orgasm to fertilize her eggs—so why (in the biological sense) does she have them at all?

Until very recently, the prevailing theory was that female orgasm did somehow offer an evolutionary advantage. Scientists assumed a link between orgasm and reproductive success, positing, for example, that orgasm aided fertilization by helping draw sperm up through the cervix and into the uterus. A dissenting opinion was first expressed by anthropologist Donald Symons in 1979. He concluded that female orgasm was simply a by-product of male orgasm (because both sexes develop from a common embryo plan). In other words, orgasm is only possible in women because it's necessary in men. Scientists didn't like that. Nor did feminists. (And get used to it: Theories about female orgasm are always put through a politically correct filter.)

Elizabeth Lloyd's 2006 book *The Case of the Female Orgasm* is an erudite and enlightened argument against all the adaptive biology theories. Yes, female orgasm is a by-product, she says, and not necessary to the procreation of the species. But the clitoris and sexual pleasure do serve an evolutionary purpose: They encourage women to have sex and thus get pregnant.

REAL TALK

Describe the best orgasm you've ever had.

"Colors! Red and pink and coral. I saw colors and flashing lights. My body was rocking and rolling like it always does, but for some reason, on that particular night, I saw colors, too."
—**Adrienne, 42**

———•———

"The first time I came during intercourse was with my husband a few months after the wedding. I was so hot for him that day. It was that time in my hormonal cycle. He picked me up at work with the top down. And he had one hand up my skirt all the way home. I was so used to not coming during intercourse that it shocked the hell out of me. It felt wonderful. All that explosion and him inside me, too."
—**Monique, 31**

———•———

"Oh, I've had so many best orgasms! I always think the one I'm having is the best."
—**Sharon, 55**

———•———

"The first one. I masturbated myself to orgasm the first time when I was 15. Wow! What a feeling. I felt myself pulsating and throbbing and I thought—this is amazing."
—**Christa, 24**

What Is an Orgasm?

In lay terms, an orgasm is generally defined as an intense, pleasurable response to genital stimulation, a release of sexual tension marked by a series of genital contractions and the release throughout the body of natural chemicals that create feelings of euphoria and attachment.

Scientists say it a bit differently:

- "The expulsive discharge of neuromuscular tensions at the peak of sexual response." –Kinsey, 1953

- "A brief episode of physical release from the vaso-congestion and myotonic increment developed in response to sexual stimuli." –Masters and Johnson, 1966

- "The zenith of sexuoerotic experience that men and women characterize subjectively as voluptuous rapture or ecstasy. It occurs simultaneously in the brain/mind and the pelvic genitalia." –Money, Wainwright, and Hingburger, 1991

TIP

———— • ————

There is a type of female orgasm rarely discussed. Betty Dodson in her book *Orgasms for Two* defines it as a "pressure orgasm." The orgasm results from indirect stimulation, or "pressure," to the clitoris and surrounding area. Some women get there by squeezing their legs together as they contract the PC muscle. Others rub back and forth against something hard like a padded headboard or chair arm. And some straddle a folded bath towel and work that back and forth between their legs, again while squeezing the PC.

" The female orgasm is one of the last frontiers of sexuality. In general, the average person knows less about the female orgasm — its causes, frequency, locations—than any other aspect of sex. "

—**Lou Paget**, American sex expert, *The Big O*

Why Does It Feel So Good?

When a woman is aroused, blood flow increases to the vagina, swelling the inner and outer lips and the clitoris. With enough intense physical and psychological stimulation, she will reach climax, during which the vagina, sphincter, and uterus contract simultaneously, and the blood congested in the vaginal area suddenly rushes back to the rest of the body. And that expulsion of tension and blood flow feels good.

Chemicals released in the brain do the rest of the feel-good work. Endorphins ease pain and elevate the sense of overall well-being. Oxytocin, a sex chemical, encourages those warm feelings of affection for her partner in orgasm. (And no big surprise: Women produce more of the "cuddly chemical" than men do.)

That chemical cocktail is most potent in the early stages of a relationship. It's called NRE, new relationship energy. Lasting anywhere from eighteen months to three years, NRE propels us into commitment, monogamy, and marriage—life choices we may begin to question when the drug wears off.

Nan Wise, "The Love Coach," has developed a tool for understanding and managing desire; she calls it the Desire Curve. We all have a Desire Set Point, the level of sexual craving we naturally feel whether in a relationship or not. In a new relationship, the level curves up and plateaus, as noted previously, for up to three years. Wise calls this period New Relationship Euphoria, or NREU. From this long high, we all go back to the Desire Set Point. (In other words, Hot Monogamy is a lie.) And some people dip past the set point into Low Desire Syndrome.

Sexually skilled lovers, however, can manage their Desire Curves by creating peaks in the valleys of their set points. For them, intersecting Desire Curves can rise and fall like waves. Wise calls the ability to do this Operational Intelligence.

"We can't really explain how arousal feels, what an orgasm is, and the closer we get to one, the less value words have, the less we can use language at all."

—**Sallie Tisdale**, *Talk Dirty to Me: An Intimate Philosophy of Sex*

What Are the Kinds of Orgasm?

For many decades, female orgasm was defined as either/or: clitoral or vaginal.

Sigmund Freud labeled clitoral orgasms as "immature" and "neurotic." The adolescent girl, he explained, experienced clitoral orgasm during masturbation. Once she became sexually active with a partner, she switched to vaginal, or "mature," orgasms. The first shrink clearly knew little about female anatomy.

In 1953, Alfred Kinsey in his landmark study, *Sexual Behavior in the Human Female*, said that all female orgasms were achieved by clitoral stimulation, either direct or indirect. His findings were endorsed a decade later by pioneer sex researchers William Masters and Virginia Johnson, who isolated the orgasm in the lab and measured and quantified the process. The clitoral orgasm theory became the prevailing opinion among sex therapists until 1980, when Beverly Whipple and John Perry claimed their research proved the existence of the G-spot, putting the origin for the female orgasm back inside the vagina.

There has not been uniform acceptance of the G-spot theory. The late Helen Singer Kaplan, Ph.D., a pioneer in sex therapy and founder of the nation's first clinic for sexual disorders, insisted that 75 percent of women do not reach orgasm without some kind of direct clitoral stimulation. Many studies reported in scientific journals have consistently reported that 60 to 75 percent of women do not reach orgasm without clitoral stimulation, with less than 10 percent of women reporting in most studies that they could, in fact, find their G-spots.

What can we learn from all this? Well, Freud was dead wrong. Kinsey and Masters and Johnson did women a great service in promoting the power of the clitoris. And if you can find your G-spot, enjoy it. If you can't, c'est la vie.

A popular theory among sex authorities now is that women can reach orgasm in a variety of ways. Try them all and see what works for you. But remember: There is no right or wrong way to come.

The orgasm routes are as follows:

Clitoral

The clitoris is rich in nerve endings, with more of them concentrated in that little organ than in the male penis. The clitoris is the only part of the body, male or female, designed purely for pleasure. Yes, the overwhelming majority of women do have clitoral orgasms.

Vaginal/Cervix

This is the orgasm that every woman seems to want, the product of deep penetration, probably by a larger than average penis. Positions that favor this type of orgasm include the woman on top and rear entry. You are more likely to experience vaginal/cervix orgasm if your clitoris lies deep inside its hood and/or you don't begin intercourse until you are on the point of orgasm and you use your PC muscle while he's thrusting.

Vaginal/G-spot

First, try to reach orgasm with a G-spot vibrator. That will show you where your G-spot is and how much stimulation it needs for orgasm. During intercourse, get into the woman-on-top position and lean back. Experiment with different angles until you feel the G-spot responding. (And play with your clitoris if you aren't getting what you need from the G-spot.)

Anal

Anal play is highly pleasurable for many women (and men), and some women do reach orgasm this way. The secrets to satisfaction? Your lover should spend a lot of time relaxing the anus, via licking and/or inserting well-lubed fingers and gently massaging. Just be sure to use lots of lube! (See more on anal sex in Chapter 10.)

Extra-genital

Some women can reach orgasm simply by having their breasts or nipples (or inner thighs or other sensitive areas) stimulated. This is most likely to happen after she has reached already orgasm once via other routes.

Blended

Some women say that their best orgasms come when two areas are being stimulated simultaneously, for example, the clitoris and vagina or anus. It's possible that some orgasms reported as vaginal or anal are really blended. If you're stroking your clitoris while you're coming from another form of stimulation, it's a blended orgasm.

Educated Women with Money Are More Likely to Orgasm

According to a joint study conducted by researchers at Sussex University and the Universities of Sydney and Melbourne, Australia, women who have "higher household income" and a "managerial/professional occupation" were most likely to reach orgasm in their sexual encounters. The study concluded that these women were more likely to have male partners who performed cunnilingus and/or to have female partners. Women who used sex toys were also "significantly more likely" to orgasm.

What does not affect orgasm potential? The age at which participants became sexually active, the number of sexual partners they had, and whether they watched Internet sex or X-rated videos.

"There is no one way to experience orgasm. The way you experience that level of sexual pleasure is as individual as you are. So experiment, keep an open mind, and enjoy your research."

—**Hilda Hutcherson, M.D.,** *Pleasure: A Woman's Guide to Getting the Sex You Want, Need, and Deserve*

To find the G-spot during intercourse, get into the woman-on-top position and lean back. Experiment with different angles until you feel it responding.

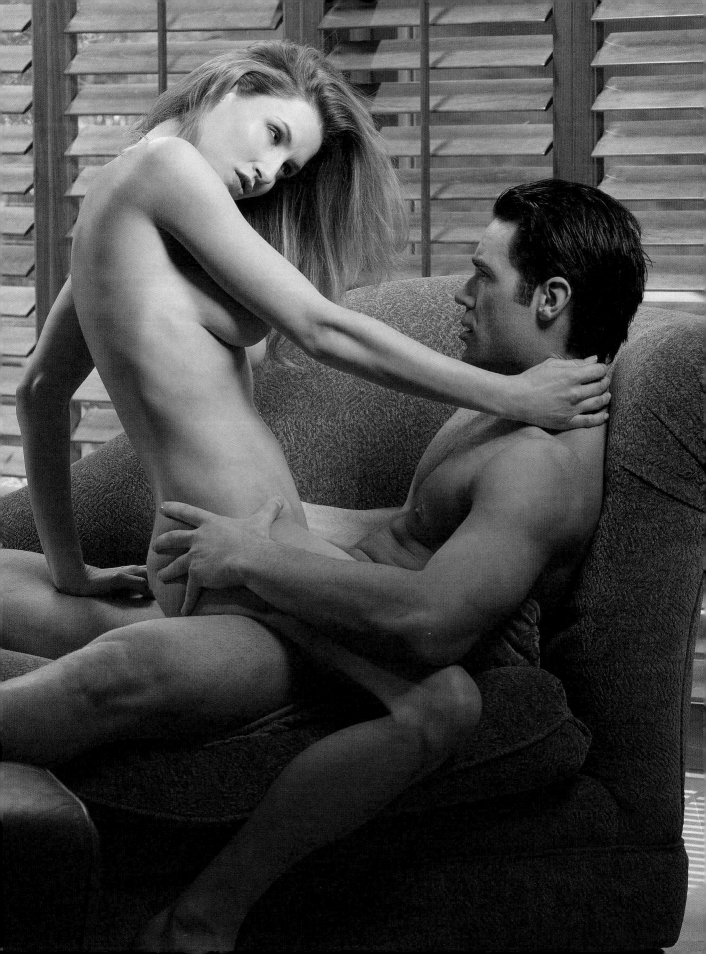

Why Do Some Women Come More Easily Than Others?

"More easily" usually means that they come during intercourse alone, because almost all women come during masturbation. The ability—or luck—to do so during intercourse is rare enough to qualify as "not the norm," yet we continue to hold up the model of female orgasm via intercourse alone as the "norm" or "ideal." That isn't fair to women or to men who blame themselves for not being able to "make" her come.

Theories about why some women orgasm more easily than others usually come down to these two: She has a larger than average clitoris or her clitoris is located deeper inside the clitoral hood, making it more likely that she gets the clitoral stimulation she needs for orgasm during intercourse alone.

From my own extensive interviews of thousands of women over two decades, I believe that location, location, location is the answer. (However, many women who say they have a large or prominent clitoris also say they cannot come during intercourse alone.) Think of the clitoris as real estate you inherited.

"What definition of 'normal' could possibly justify labeling two-thirds of women as 'abnormal'?"

—Elisabeth Lloyd, *The Case of the Female Orgasm*, challenging the popular (and therapeutically accepted) belief that the failure to achieve orgasm is a female sexual dysfunction

"Do yourself and him a favor, sister: Fake it. If you are happy and generous—minded, you will fake it and then leap out of bed and make breakfast, squeeze orange juice or pour Champagne, telling him, 'You are so clever,' or however you express enthusiasm."

—**Fay Weldon**, controversial British feminist author, *What Makes Women Happy*

Faking!

The advice to "fake it" may be the common wisdom, but it's terrible advice. Statistics from women's magazine surveys to research conduced by university psychology departments report that women do fake orgasm, and in consistently high numbers. Would you believe that 85 percent of women have faked an orgasm at least once in their lives? (And the other 15 percent are either virgins or liars.)

The biggest reason not to fake it is that you're saying, "Honey, that worked!," but it didn't. It won't work next time, either. Faking may end the sex, but it isn't going to make you happy.

I am not encouraging you to criticize his technique or blame him for not pleasing you. Ask for what you want and need in the moment, not later. Learn how to have an orgasm. And then make sure you do have them.

TIP

If you're going to fake it for whatever reason, don't go over the top. Women who fake typically over-emote. (Apparently even this does fool many men, though.) A more discerning male lover, however, will get suspicious if you shout, scream, gasp, and pant like a porn actress. Take the performance down a notch or two. And afterward, don't leap out of bed or launch into conversation. Authentic orgasm does leave a woman a little breathless and somewhat speechless for a few or several minutes.

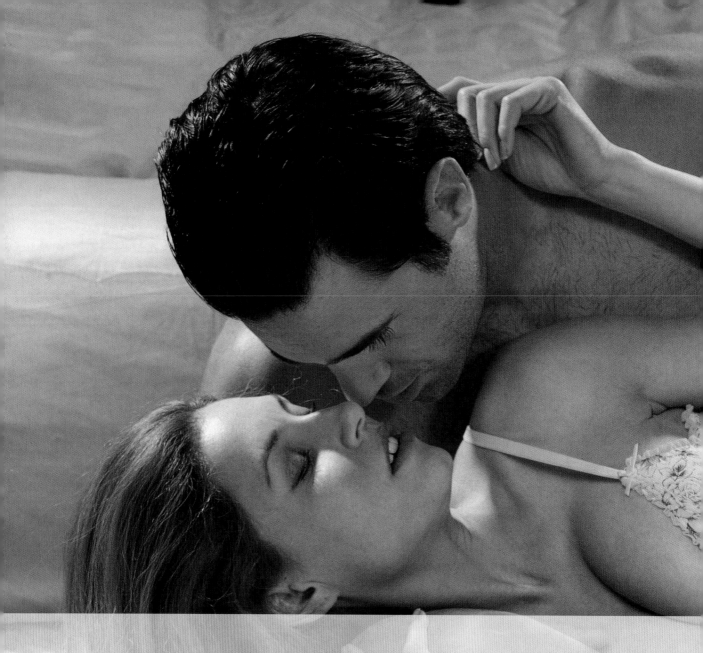

Chapter 9

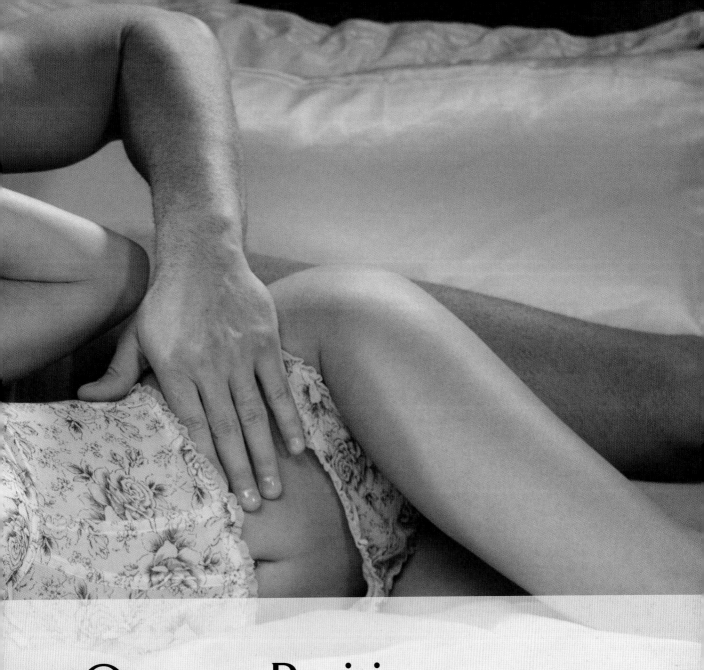

Orgasm Positions

Let's not call them "intercourse positions." I'd rather you think more positively. These are orgasm positions because you can have an orgasm in any one of them, even if your hot spots don't connect. You can use your hand or a finger vibe or delay intercourse until you are seconds away from coming. Any position is an orgasm position.

And you will finally get the answer to that question: "How can I come during intercourse?"

TIP

— • —

Is there a best position for female orgasm? Yes—any one of them. The female superior, or woman-on-top, position is usually touted as the "best" position for her orgasm. But a woman who isn't comfortable on top won't make it work to her advantage because she won't touch herself. Any position can become your own "best." Everything depends on how your bodies fit together and how you adapt that position to get the maximum clitoral benefits.

Another trick to finding your personal best is asking yourself: In what position can I most effectively contract and release the PC muscle during thrusting? For some women, that is missionary position with your feet pressed against his chest. Try it and see how it works for you.

The Key to Reaching Orgasm

When a woman says, "I can't come with him," she usually means: "I can't come with any man during intercourse alone." That's normal. You realize that now, right? Stop faking. Whether you reach orgasm or you don't has little to do with him and much to do with you.

Here's how to reach orgasm with your partner:

Manual Stimulation During Intercourse, in Any Position

Either of you has to touch the clitoris and the surrounding tissue during intercourse, or you should bring a vibe to bed with you.

One or the other needs only to insert a finger or two down below, between your bodies, and stroke. If you're too shy to touch yourself in front of him or to tell him how you like to be touched, just take his hand, put it there, and move against it.

Or one of you can use a finger vibe. Or you can wear a strap-on vibe. Or you must masturbate to the point where orgasm is imminent before intercourse. Or he must arouse you to fever pitch via manual and/or oral stimulation before intercourse begins. At that point, any movement in the genital area should put you over the edge, especially if you have a strong PC muscle and flex like mad.

Really, isn't this easy? Why make it difficult?

The Flying V

Now that you're getting over your shyness about needing clitoral stimulation, or your reluctance to accept the obvious—that most women don't come via intercourse alone—here's a simple move that can really take you where you want to go, in any intercourse position.

Many women find this simple move more effective for inducing orgasm than directly stroking or circling the clitoris, especially during intercourse, when the space available between bodies does limit the options a bit.

Insert two fingers of one hand between your bodies. Form a V shape with your fingers, straddling your clitoris. Push the V down in time with his thrusting.

Or take his fingers and place them in the V shape on the sides of your clitoris. Grind against his fingers as he thrusts.

TIP

—— · ——

Your favorite orgasm position not working as well as it used to? Bodies change. Weight gain or loss, athletic injuries, a subtle decline in erectile function, and other factors can make a difference. Try some of the adaptations under The Basic Six Positions (at right). And experiment with new ones.

The Basic Six Positions

There are six basic intercourse positions and, of course, numerous variations to each of them.

They are:

- Woman on top (or female superior)
- Man on top (or missionary)
- Side-by-side
- Rear entry
- Sitting
- Standing

Female Superior Position

Considered by sex therapists and women who respond to reader surveys to be the intercourse position most conducive to female orgasm, the woman-on-top position is also a favorite of men. (They like to watch.) She can easily reach her clitoris and she controls the depth, angle, and speed of thrusting. In the most common variation of the position, she squats or sits astride (in a riding position) the man, who is lying on his back.

She may lean forward, putting her weight on her hands on either side of his shoulders, or she may lean on one hand, or maintain an upright position, keeping both hands free. She may also lean backward, if that gives her better G-spot stimulation. A common variation on the position is the "reverse cowgirl," where she faces his feet, not his head.

Better Orgasms in This Position

Here's how to make it an even better orgasm position:

- Alternate deep thrusting with using the head of his penis to stimulate your clitoris.

- Move from side to side rather than up and down.

- When orgasm is imminent, flatten yourself out on top of him, clench your thighs together, and grind your clitoris into him as you flex your PC muscle.

- In the reverse cowgirl, ask him to raise one leg and place his foot on the bed. Angle your body so that you are riding his penis at the same time you're grinding against his raised thigh.

The Oval Track

Use this sizzling move in the female superior position. It looks as good to him as it feels to you.

Simply move in an oval track rather than a straight-forward up-and-down riding motion. Imagine you are circumscribing an oval with your body, with the down-stroke at one end of the oval and the upstroke at the other. Lean slightly forward as you push down on his penis, stimulating your clitoris. Pull up and move slightly backward on the upstroke, stimulating your G-spot.

And, of course, use your hand if you need it. And flex that PC muscle!

REAL TALK

What's your favorite position for female orgasm?

"Rear entry. I love to look at a woman's ass. And the power! I bring her to the edge of the bed and I stand behind her and take her and she is completely mine—and I know she is comin'."
—Ahmed, 29

———•———

"Right now with this guy, it's the good old missionary. We are athletic with it, moving it around to get what I need. I like wrapping my legs around his neck or putting my feet on his chest. With other guys, it's been other favorite positions."
—Nadine, 36

———•———

"Rear entry. I love the way my guy pounds my pussy in that position. Sometimes it's just what I crave. And it's easier for me to play with my clit if he's not looking right at me while I do it."
—Marisol, 30

———•———

"My favorite position is me on top. I'm a bit of an exhibitionist. And I know I look good riding my man. I can work my G-spot and get clit play. It has everything. And he doesn't seem to mind that it's my favorite."
—Amelia, 44

———•———

"It's all good. When I want to make up to her for working late or ignoring her to watch sports on TV, I start out on top of her, then roll her to the side while I'm still in her and hold her really close in what I call 'the package.' I have my leg wrapped around her ass and my arm around her back and I'm saying, 'I love you, baby, you're the one.'"
—Tyrone, 39

Experiment with different variations of the female superior position. Have him sit up to kiss and hold you, for example.

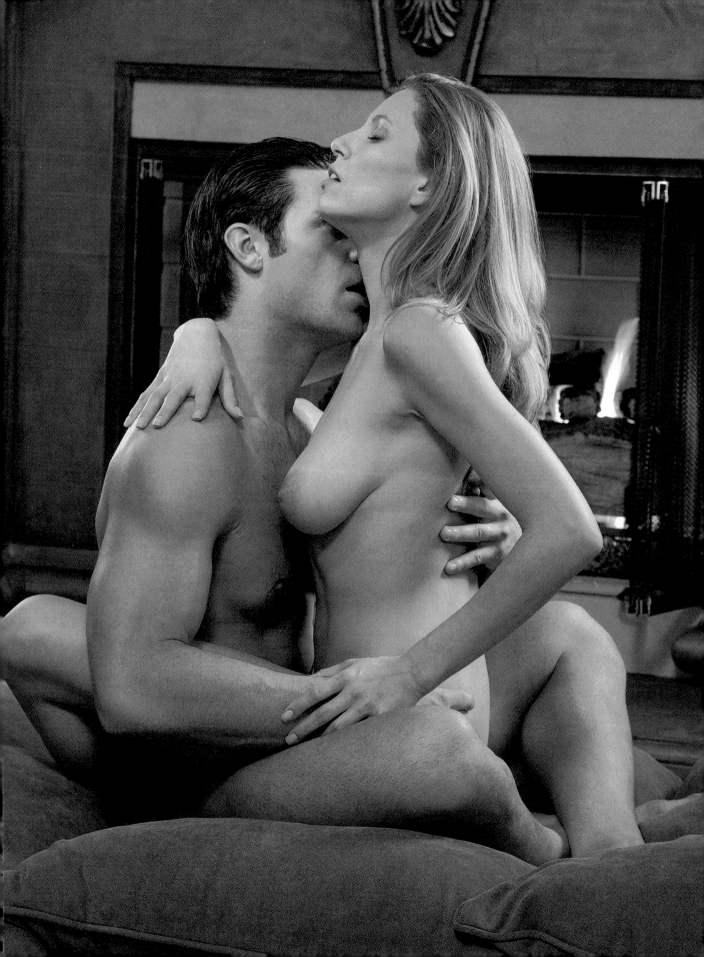

Missionary Position

In surveys, women usually rate this position more favorably than men do, probably because it allows for hard thrusting. And, yes, women like that!

In the most common variation of the position, she lies on her back with her legs slightly parted and he lies on top of her, supporting himself at least partially with his hands.

Better Orgasms in This Position

Here's how to make it a better orgasm position:

- Place a pillow(s) beneath the small of your back to change the angle of penetration to one of greater depth.

- Lie on your back with your legs up as straight and high as they will comfortably go. He kneels in front of you. This tightens your vagina, providing greater friction for both of you, and it leaves your hands free to play with your clitoris.

- Lie on your back and put your legs over his shoulders.

- Lift one leg up and put it over his shoulder or around his back.

- Put your feet on his chest or shoulders, again to change the angle of penetration and control the thrust.

- Wrap your legs around his waist or his neck for the same reasons.

- Pull her to the edge of the bed. He either holds her legs or she wraps them around him as he enters her from a standing position.

New Man on Top

This position offers maximum sensation for her with minimal movement for him, and it can help sustain intercourse longer.

She lies on her stomach, legs straight out and spread only slightly. He lies over her, supporting his weight on his elbows. He positions his legs on either side of her. As he enters her, she closes her legs and crosses them at the ankles.

Crossing your ankles and holding your legs together enables you to feel the entire length of his penis inside you. As he is thrusting, he's in a great position to kiss your neck and nibble your ears. And you can reach under and play with your clitoris.

It's new, it's fun, and it works.

" Missionary is the do-me position. And I am a do-me girl in bed."

–Female CEO, 39

Side-by-Side Position

Often a favorite position for the weary couple—or the semi-erect man—side-by-side is sometimes called "spooning" and even "stuffing and spooning."

In the basic version of the position, he faces her back. Her buttocks are angled against him as he puts one leg between hers. Or she can lie half on her back, half on her side, drawing up the leg upon which she is lying. He faces her.

Variations

They can face one another, with legs loosely wrapped around each other. Or they can keep their legs touching and out straight—with the other legs loosely wrapped.

In another variation, they face one another and she wraps both legs around him—like a lying-down version of stand-up sex.

Better Orgasms in This Position

Here's how to make it a better orgasm position:

- Either you or he stimulates your clitoris.

- Add a vibrator. This is a great position for vibe play because your hands are free.

- Make this your go-to position when he is tired, but you want sex. Masturbate first until you are highly aroused. He will feel good that he is able to "give" you an orgasm.

Rear-Entry Position

A favorite position of the ancient Chinese, rear entry is also a favorite of both sexes in the West today, in spite of its unfortunate nickname, "doggy style." This position facilitates deep penetration, G-spot stimulation, and hard thrusting, and puts her clitoris in a good place for manual stimulation. A nice bonus: Her ass looks its best here, with the little wrinkles and pockets fairly well ironed out. (Who doesn't love that?)

In the basic position, the woman is on all fours with the man kneeling behind her.

Variations

He stands behind her and pulls her to the edge of the bed. Standing gives him the ability to thrust even more forcefully—something both partners may want.

In another variation, she lowers her chest to the bed. That changes the angle of penetration. Some women report greater G-spot stimulation in this variation.

Better Orgasms in This Position

Here's how to make it better for orgasm:

- Lower your upper body so that your chest touches the bed. This elongates your vaginal barrel, making a "tighter" fit for his penis.

- If he typically grabs your hips or ass and controls the thrusting, ask him to caress your vulva and finger your clitoris while otherwise remaining relatively still while you thrust back against him.

- Try rear entry lying down, with you on your stomach. Clench your thighs together after he enters you and lift one leg for deeper penetration.

The Sitting Position

There's a lot you can do with this one because it works with different levels of passion. It's good if he's tired or you feel like talking and playing. But it's also good when you just have to sit on him now.

In the basic position, he sits in a chair or on the bed with her astride him. Penetration is shallow.

Variations

Changing the chair also changes the angle and depth of penetration—and her ability to leverage thrusting. A hard-backed kitchen chair, for example, gives her thrusting power, while an overstuffed chair may not.

She sits on him, facing away from him. Again, that changes the angle and depth of penetration.

Better Orgasms in This Position

Here's how to make it a better position for orgasm:

- He grasps your buttocks firmly, and you lean backward as he thrusts.

- Add a vibrator, especially a vibrating cock ring on him or a strap-on vibe for you.

- Sit on the kitchen counter, washer or dryer, or a high bar stool—whatever is the right height for him to enter you.

"It's a myth that women don't like rear entry. We do like vigorous thrusting. And we don't always need to see your face."

–Kate, sex researcher

Try combining the sitting and standing positions by having the man sit back on the edge of chair. The woman can also use the chair to maneuver herself onto him.

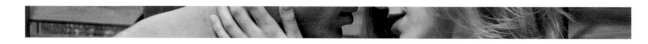

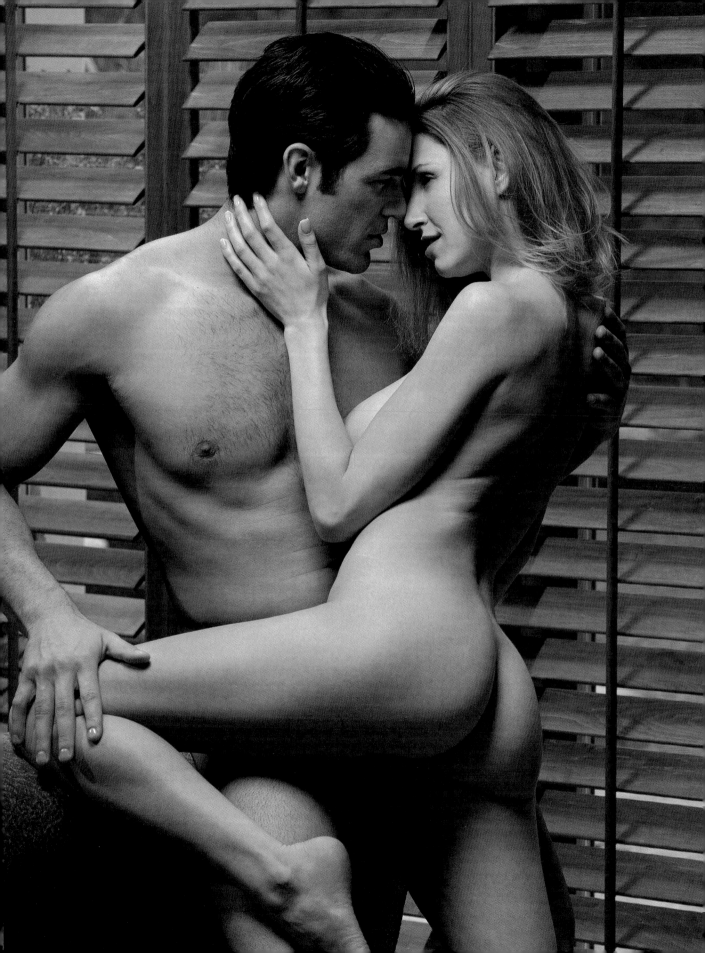

The Standing Position

Having intercourse while standing satisfies a need we all have sometimes for dramatic, urgent lovemaking. It's a great way to have a quickie or to begin a longer session. You can always slide to the floor and finish in another position.

In the basic version of the position, he squats slightly while she lowers herself onto him. She wraps one leg around his waist and he holds her buttocks.

Variations

This might be "cheating," but he can lift her onto a kitchen counter, washer or dryer, or any convenient surface when standing becomes uncomfortable.

"Many women say they cannot have sex standing up. Many women say they cannot have an orgasm with a man on top. Many women say they have their best orgasms with him on top. Many women are not in your bed. Nevermind what they say. What works for you?"

–iVillage.com

Better Orgasms in This Position

Here's how to make it better for orgasm:

- Change the depth and angle of penetration by doing it on the stairs, with you one step above him.

- You stand in front of him, facing in the opposite direction. Bend slightly forward. You'll feel more G-spot stimulation this way.

TIP

——•——

Sometimes you want to make love like a porn star. Try the standing position in front of a full length mirror. Use props—like a sturdy barstool than he can lean back against—if a wall isn't handy. This can be especially effective as a visual treat if a mini skirt is pulled up to her waist, exposing her buttocks.

The standing position is great if you're looking for quick satisfaction or a change from your horizontal routine.

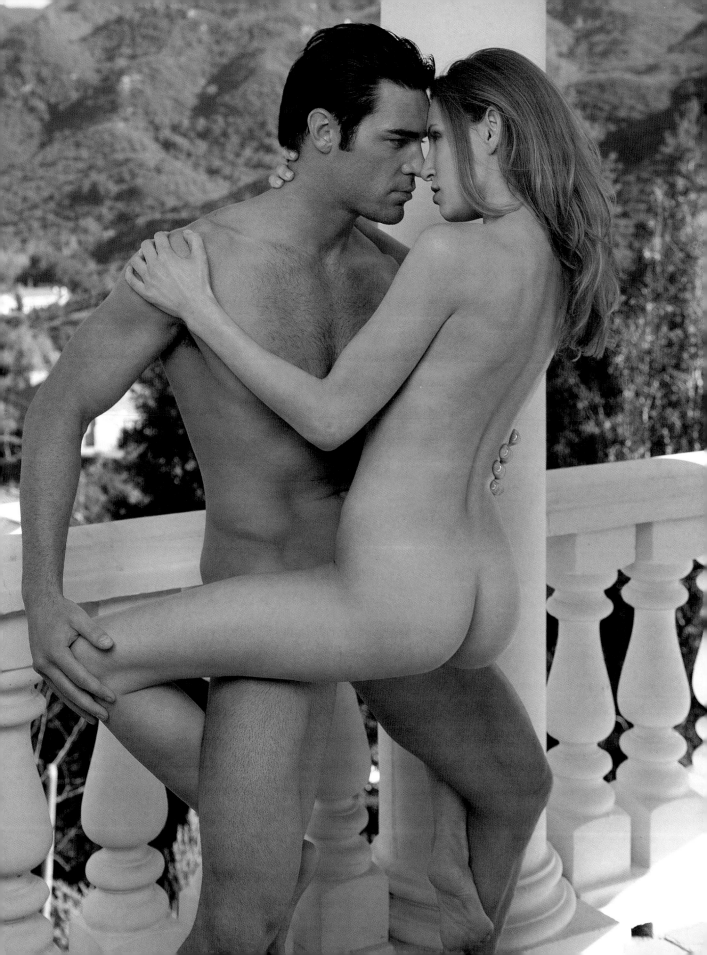

Chapter 10

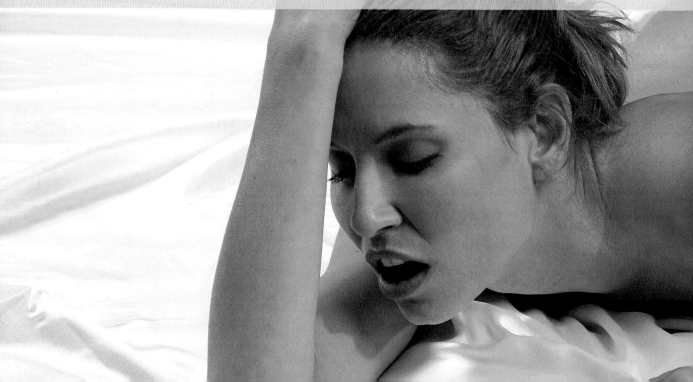

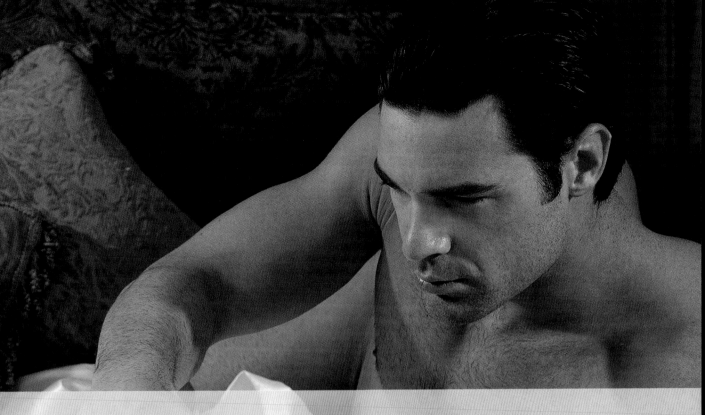

Quickies, Anal Orgasms, and Multiples

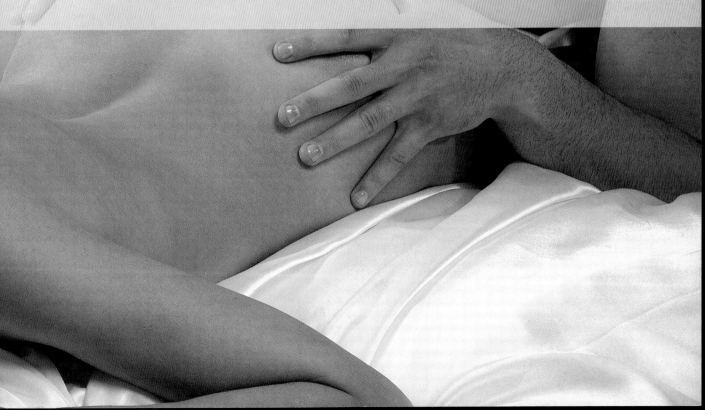

This is the place to let go of some of your assumptions about orgasm.

- Do you think quickies are something women do for men—because she won't come but he will?

- Do you believe that anal orgasms are myths—maybe myths perpetrated by husbands who want anal sex?

- Do you suspect that multiple orgasms are the figment of sex journalists' imaginations?

All these things—and more—will be sorted out and put to rest in this chapter.

"Why quick sex? Because it just might save your sex life."

—**Tracey Cox**, British sex expert, *Quickies*

REAL TALK

Where is the most public place you've had sex?

"On the steps of the Lincoln Memorial in Washington, D.C. My lover was with the State Department, and we got out of his government car to walk around the mall. The driver was parked and waiting for us. My lover sat down on the steps, and pulled me onto his lap. One thing led to another. And I wasn't wearing panties."
—**Susannah, 45**

—— • ——

"In a Holiday Inn swimming pool outside St. Louis. I was in town for a cousin's wedding. The wedding party stayed at the hotel. The reception was winding down when one of the bridesmaids took my hand and suggested a walk. We saw the empty pool, stripped down, jumped in, and fucked like water bunnies. Later I learned that she had a thing for the groom."
—**Joe, 32**

—— • ——

"I was having a late lunch with a guy pal at a trendy Soho [New York City] restaurant two days before Christmas. My flight to the West Coast had been cancelled due to a snowstorm. He was Jewish and going through a divorce. So we were both alone for the day, expected nowhere. We drank a lot of wine. The restaurant was empty. We were kissing and groping . . . and suddenly I decided to get under the table and blow him. Then he did me. We left a 200 percent tip."
—**Ingrid, 40**

How to Make a Quickie Work for Her, Too

There isn't always time for the kind of extended foreplay and long lovemaking sessions that favor women's orgasms. Modern couples, especially two-career plus kids couples, don't have that kind of time every day, or even most days. They put sex off 'til Saturday night. Maybe they even avoid touching one another in bed because they don't want to start something that one or both has neither the time nor the energy to finish. The weekend comes and someone has a cold, the in-laws are visiting, social obligations have piled up. Soon sex avoidance becomes a habit. Before they know what has happened to them, they become that couple who can't remember the last time they had sex.

Unless you have the luxury of time every day of the week, you need to learn the art of the quickie. Sex begets sex. The more you have, the more you want. The less you have—well, you don't want to go there, do you?

Myths and Misconceptions of Quickies

Keep the following myths in mind; remember, these are not true:

- Women can't come during a quickie.

- If you let a man "have" a quickie, he won't want to do it any other way.

- Only couples that are new to each other have the kind of passionate desire that fuels a quickie.

- It's over before she's had a chance to lubricate.

- A quickie is just another name for "premature-ejaculation sex."

"Women who have a strong PC muscle not only experience more pleasure in sex and have more frequent orgasms—they are far more likely to reach orgasm in a quickie."

—**Hilda Hutcherson, M.D.**, author and *Glamour* magazine columnist

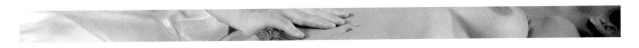

The Quickie Essentials

Want a quickie to work for both of you? Here are some tips:

Sex your brain: Sure, it's possible that lust takes you by surprise. You get swept up in passion. You melt at the sight of him. You grow erect when she unbuttons her blouse. But if you can't wait for lust to take you like a pirate swooping up booty, then encourage your sexual thoughts and fantasies, especially just before you'll have time for a quickie. Put sex in your head. Pretend you are meeting your lover in an empty conference room and time is of the essence.

Prepare your body: Use a lube like Liquid Silk or the new KY vaginal moisturizer that you can put in a little ahead of time. She can use a Pocket Rocket vibe to rev up. In less than two minutes, she'll be ready. And always wear lingerie that can pushed aside. No pantyhose!

Redefine sex: "Sex" doesn't have to mean intercourse. A Quickie could be mutual oral sex in the back seat of the car parked in the garage while the kids are watching *The Little Mermaid* inside the house. You can skip the foreplay this time. Really. If she's lubed and revved up and he has an erection, you're good to go. Intercourse in a standing position, sitting on his lap in a chair, or in a position that would be uncomfortable for long play adds a sense of urgency and excitement to the event.

Touch her clitoris: Use your hand or a finger vibe, but don't neglect clitoral stimulation.

Be edgy: Do it in the backyard at midnight, the restroom of your favorite pub, your mother's gazebo—there are so many places to have a quickie, especially since you don't take all your clothes off. The risk of being seen also adds an element of excitement.

"Do you know what I love about a quickie? Even if you're in a relationship, it's not about the relationship."

—**Parker Posey**, Indie film star

TIP

Don't put pressure on the quickie. Enjoy it for the lusty, dramatic experience that it is. Orgasm will most likely be part of the experience if you're using the Orgasm Loop (see Chapter 11). But if it doesn't happen, masturbate after he leaves (or falls asleep). Let the quickie be the one "no expectations" sexual event in your sex life.

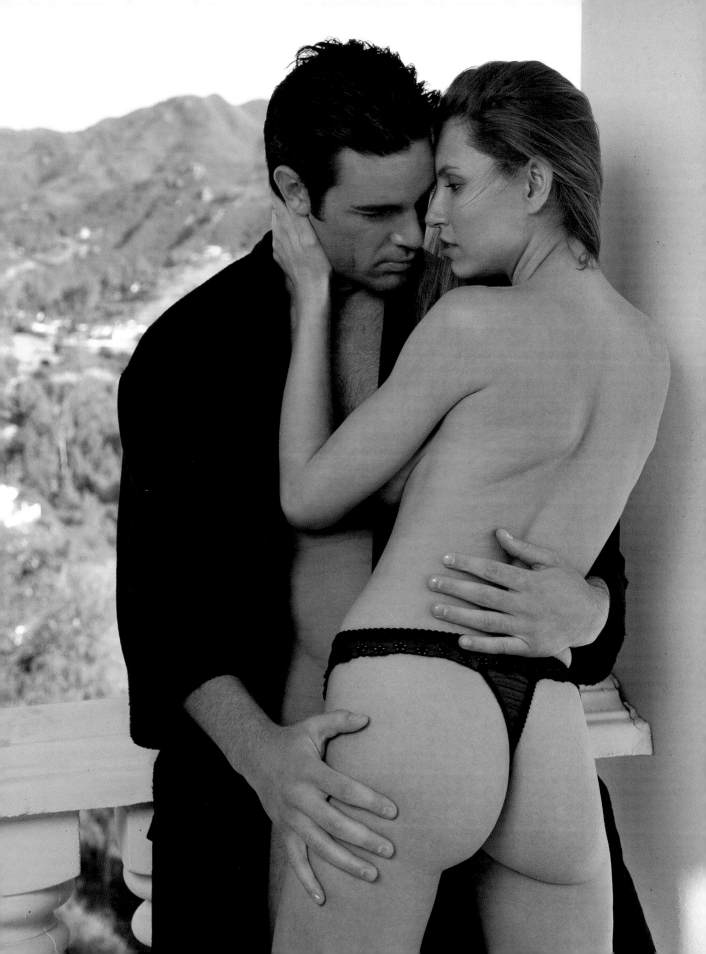

Anal Intercourse

Anal? Really? Really. The anal orgasm is not just a theory promulgated by men trying to get women to try anal intercourse. The anus, in both sexes, is rich in nerve endings. Stimulating it does bring pleasure.

Bring on the toys, fingers, and tongues, and see whether anal play arouses you before trying anal intercourse.

Anal Massage

- Massage her buttocks using firm strokes. Then use light, teasing strokes—even gentle pinching—down the crack between her cheeks.

- Separating the buttocks slightly, massage the innermost parts with somewhat gentler strokes than you used on the outer buttocks.

- Apply the light, teasing strokes you used in her crack down to her anus. With a well-lubed finger, circle the anal opening lightly.

- Using long strokes, begin massaging her buttocks again, starting at the base of the spine and continuing down the perineum.

- Massage her perineum with your thumb or finger pad, exerting light pressure.

- Put your finger in her anus and gently circle inside the opening. Now add a second finger. Rub them in and out in simulated intercourse. (She can do all this to him, too.)

Anal Toys

Consider using the following anal toys:

- **Anal beads:** Made of jelly, plastic, or silicone, anal beads look like the necklaces made of pop beads that you had as a child. At the end of this string of beads is a large circular pull. You gently insert the (well-lubricated) beads, then pull them out, one bead at a time, for an ooh-la-la effect. Flexi Felix, made of silicone, is a high-quality product, with no rough edges on the beads, and it is easier to clean than the cheap versions.

- **Butt plugs:** Varying in size and somewhat in shape, butt plugs are insertable wands that have a flared base so you don't have to worry about them getting lost up there. Used during masturbation, they will make you aware that your anal muscles really do clench in orgasm—and they will heighten the sensation of that. As preparation for anal sex, a butt plug opens the pathway. Some women find that using a butt plug during intercourse gives them a delicious feeling of double penetration and expands their orgasm. Use lots of lube. (And if he wants you to try a butt plug, why don't you ask him to try one, too?)

- **Anal vibrators or attachments:** Anal vibrators are specially designed for anal insertion. They are smaller—both shorter and thinner—than regular vibes.

Sex play before anal intercourse should include everything you like—cunnilingus, probably to orgasm, manual clitoral stimulation, a lot of kissing and caressing, and, of course, anal play.

Anal Intercourse

Before beginning, get the necessary props:

- A good lubricant, such as Astroglide (no scented oils, lotions, or petroleum jelly)

- An anal condom, necessary to keep bacteria out of his urethra

Step #1: Find the position

For men and women—especially beginners—the rear-entry position with her chest flat on the bed and ass elevated is the easiest position. There are other options, too.

For example, you can try these:

- Lie on your back with your legs straight up or your ankles resting on his shoulders while he kneels between your legs.

- In the female superior position, you lower yourself onto him while he lies on his back.

- Lower yourself onto him in the sitting position.

- Use the side-by-side position with your ass against his penis.

Step #2: Lube up

Using strokes that you find pleasurable, he generously lubes your anus and rectum.

Step #3: Start slowly

As he presses the head of his penis against your anus, relax the sphincter muscles in your rectum. Push the muscles out so that you are pushing onto him as he is pressing into you. He shouldn't force entry. Rather, you should bear down on the head of his penis until he is past the sphincter muscles.

Step #4: Begin thrusting

He begins to thrust slowly and carefully, following your lead. You control the depth and speed of penetration.

Step #5: Stimulate the clit

While he is thrusting, you (or he, but only if his fingers are clean) stimulate your clitoris.

Afterward, he must not insert his penis or fingers into your vagina until he has disposed of the condom and washed his hands. I don't mean to sound like a clean freak, but you both risk contracting a urinary tract infection from anal sex if the cleanliness rules are not followed scrupulously. No vaginal sex after anal sex until he has washed.

Remember: Porn films are vehicles for arousal, not how-to videos. So never mind that porn actors slide in and out of orifices with no time-outs for washing (and no specs of feces on their penises, either). That is not real life.

Multiple Orgasms

Theoretically, any/every woman can have multiple orgasms, because women, unlike men, do not have a refractory period following orgasm. How many women actually do report having multiple orgasms? In most surveys and studies, it is 10 percent or fewer.

Types of Multiples

There are four types of multiple orgasms:

- **Compounded single orgasms:** Each orgasm is distinct, separated by sufficient time so that prior arousal and tension have substantially resolved between orgasms.

- **Sequential multiples:** Orgasms are fairly close together—anywhere from 2 to 10 minutes apart—with little interruption in sexual stimulation or level of arousal.

- **Serial multiples:** Orgasms are separated by seconds, or up to 1 or 3 minutes, with no or barely any interruption in stimulation or diminishment of arousal.

- **Blended multiples:** A mix of two or more of the above types. Very often women who are multi-orgasmic experience more than one type of multiple orgasm during a lovemaking session.

Encouraging Multiples

What can you do to encourage multiple orgasms? Here are some tips:

- **Start on warm:** Fantasize about the sexual encounter before it begins. Masturbate, but not to orgasm. Indulge in sensual cues, such as candles, music, perfume, and lingerie. Set time aside for longer than usual lovemaking.

- **Focus:** You must be focused solely on your pleasure to achieve multiples. If you are paying too much attention to him—even to pleasing him—you won't get there. You probably won't have them if you're tired, stressed, or angry, particularly with your lover. Mental attitude is crucial. Shut out intrusive thoughts. (See Chapter 11 for advice on how to do that.)

- **Touch yourself:** A woman who has multiple orgasms is comfortable giving herself additional clitoral stimulation during sex.

What Can He Do to Help?

Unless you're masturbating to multiple orgasms, the pursuit is something of a joint effort. He won't mind at all. Men are somewhat in awe of the female ability to come and come again—and they feel like more powerful lovers if their woman does.

- **Alternate stimuli:** During lovemaking, alternate physical stimuli. The first one or two orgasms, for example, may be via cunnilingus or manual stimulation. Rarely will a woman have multiples if you move from foreplay straight to intercourse.

- **Use your hands:** Touch her clitoris. When she isn't stroking her clitoris, you probably should be. Don't leave her clitoris alone for too long if you want to help her reach orgasm multiple times. If she is G-spot responsive, use your fingers to stimulate her G-spot while you perform cunnilingus.

- **Try The Flame:** For some women, this is the ultimate cunnilingus stroke. Pretend the tip of your tongue is a candle flame. In your mind's eye, see that flame flickering in the wind. Move your tongue rapidly around the sides of her clitoris, above and below it, as the candle flame moves.

"Multiple orgasms! Any woman who has orgasms can have multiples. Few do. Most don't bother."

—**Anne Thatcher**, sex therapist

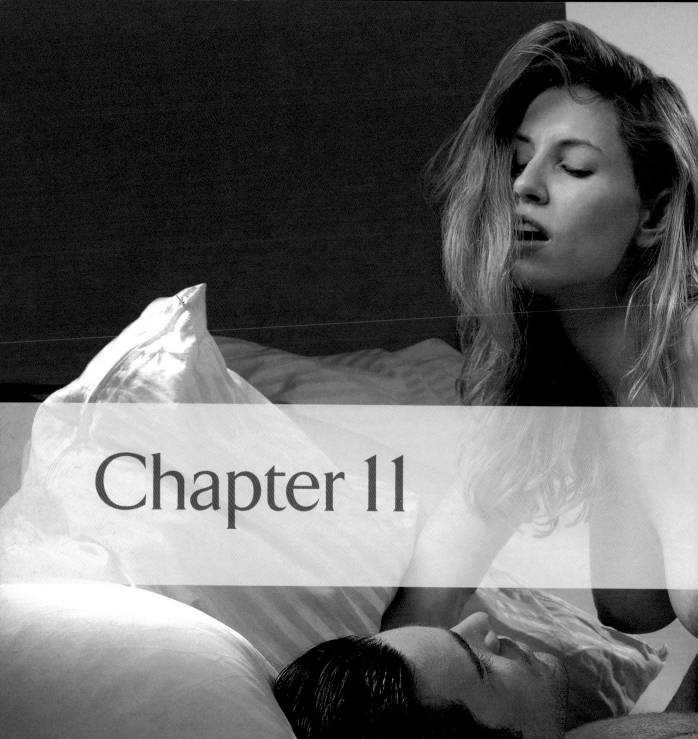

Chapter 11

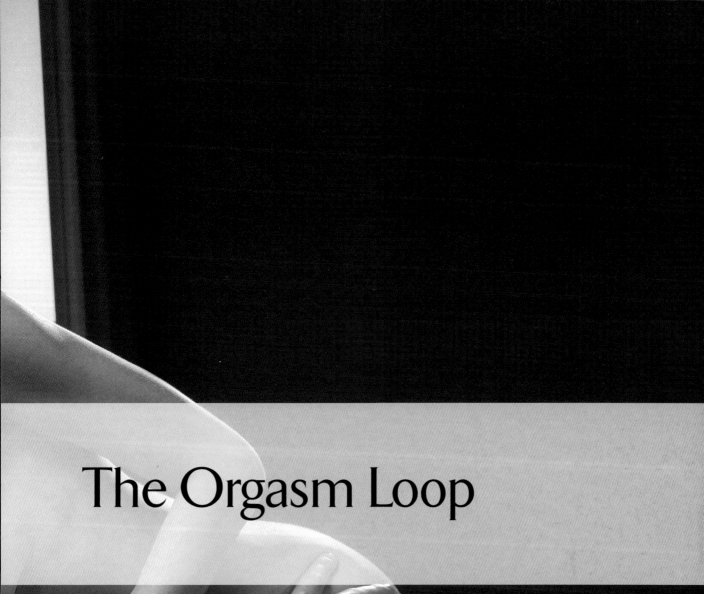

The Orgasm Loop

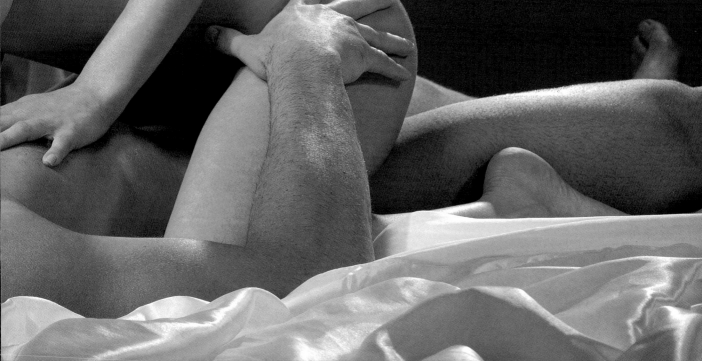

invented the Orgasm Loop (or O Loop), a revolutionary mind/body technique, in response to that question I've heard from thousands of women over the past two decades: "How can I have an orgasm during intercourse?"

I am not alone in reporting that this is indeed women's number one sex concern. Everyone who deals with female sexuality for a living knows what the question is. And we all know the simple answer.

You would be living in the woods now had not so many trees been felled in service of the answer to that question.

Perhaps a better question is, "Why don't women know how to come during intercourse?"

This is a more complex question than it appears to be. The obvious answer—and the answer I have been giving for decades!—is to touch yourself during intercourse. But this is advice some women aren't willing to hear, much less follow. (What?! And let the Prince think his magic wand isn't sufficient?)

So, I began looking for a long answer for women who just don't want the short one. Here's what I knew when I started: Women of varying ages and levels of sexual expertise have difficulty reaching orgasm with their partners, and sometimes alone. At least a third of women are reluctant to masturbate, or they do masturbate without touching themselves. (Straddling towels is surprisingly common. Yet no one writes about the problem of chafing.) While vibrators are increasingly popular sex toys, many women don't know how get the most out of them. And they complain that they either have trouble becoming aroused or sustaining arousal during lovemaking, typically citing distractions like worrying about work or domestic chores when they want to be abandoning themselves to pleasure. That arousal problem compounds their orgasm difficulties.

I then asked myself, "What if I could figure out how all women can experience the great orgasms that many women do achieve during masturbation, and transfer that thrill to lovemaking?" I began by researching techniques for removing the mental roadblocks to arousal. Once I discovered the cognitive feedback loop studies conducted by Dr. Eileen Palace at Tulane University in Louisiana (U.S.), I knew I could simplify the concept, integrate creative visualization, add some adapted sex techniques from Tantra, and take advantage of a woman's natural sexual arousal patterns. But the Orgasm Loop didn't come together until I realized one day, while talking to an old family friend in Illinois—a man with several black belts, that energy focus as practiced by experts in martial arts was the real key to the Orgasm Loop's success.

It was the most exciting moment of my professional life. I've tested it on dozens of women to date, with overwhelmingly positive results. The Orgasm Loop taps into a woman's arousal potential and teaches her how to use her body to her own best orgasmic advantage.

The first few times you use the Orgasm Loop, you'll have to think about what you're doing. You will need to focus more on achieving arousal and getting your own pleasure than on your partner. (He won't mind. The results will be worth it for both of you, because a man's number one desire is to "give" his partner an orgasm.) After that, the technique comes naturally—as, hopefully, your orgasms will.

TIP

— • —

Like so many women, do you start worrying about your orgasm shortly after the lovemaking begins? Will I—or won't I? It's the question that derails the love train. The Orgasm Loop takes the worry out of sex. You focus on arousal to the point where negative thoughts cannot intrude.

Step #1. Visualize Arousal Before You Begin Lovemaking

For women, sex definitely does begin in the mind. Like most women, you may not even know your body is aroused when it is because you won't allow yourself the time to think about sex. Give yourself that time before the foreplay begins. Slip into the bathroom, if necessary. Close your eyes, clear your mind, and visualize arousal as an image, perhaps a color like red, or a flower like an orchid, or a scene such as the beach at sunset. The secret lies in keeping the image simple, clean, and constant, so that every time you see it in your mind, you think: I am aroused. The more you use the image, the more you condition yourself to be aroused.

Some women who tested the technique asked, "Can't I make my arousal image a mental photo of my husband?"

No! The image of the man you love may call up different emotions depending on whether or not he did his share of the chores that week or any number of other factors. You need to tap into arousal as a pure force of its own volition—a force inside you—not a complicated emotion dependent on your feelings at the moment for your partner. Love is complex. Arousal is simple. You must get inside your own sexual moment before you can be a good partner to him.

An important note: If you are using this step (visualizing arousal) during foreplay with your partner, keep your eyes closed as he kisses, caresses, and strokes you, and focus on your mental arousal image. Making love with your eyes open is great—once you are fully aroused. But in this beginning state, you need to focus on your own arousal, not your intense, intimate connection with your partner.

Step # 2. Focus Energy During Foreplay

Imagine that all the energy in your body is focused in two places: one, a spot slightly below your navel, called the "inner chi" by devotees of Eastern erotic arts (because of its proximity to the genitals), and two, the spot at the base of your spine, considered the site of sexual energy by practitioners of Kundalini yoga. Imagine you are holding energy in those two places until they feel alive with sexual desire. Visualize the energy there. (Just as you can hold your leg or arm out from your body by willing those muscles to perform, you can hold your energy in place.) When you focus on the energy, you feel your body growing hotter and more desirous.

Now create a circle of fire by breathing deeply in and out and picturing your breath as fire. Move that fiery energy in a circular fashion as you draw a deep, slow breath into your nostrils and mouth. Push the fire breath down and feel it licking the base of your spine before you expel it out of your body through your genitals. Do it again. Breathe into your nostrils and mouth and out through your genitals. See your breath as a fiery circle that ignites your passion. Erotic breathing naturally turns up the sexual volume.

"The number one sex question we get from readers is, 'How can I have an orgasm during intercourse?'"

—Kate White, Editor-in-Chief, *Cosmopolitan* magazine

Step # 3. Move Your Body During Intercourse

Flex your PC muscles in time with your fire breathing. During intercourse, position yourself to make the hot spot connection (between your clitoris and/or G-spot and the head of his penis), and use your hand for extra stimulation, if necessary. That hot spot connection triggers orgasm, so use whatever position or leverage you need to get it. Because you have been concentrating so intensely on arousal and sexual energy, you will be more sensitive to erotic touch now than you usually are. You will reach orgasm quickly.

And Don't Stop

That's right . . . if you want another orgasm, don't stop.

Just don't let yourself relax into the post-orgasmic state. Stay in the Orgasm Loop by closing your eyes and going back to visualizing arousal, followed by energy focusing and fire breathing. The next orgasm—and the one after that—will follow.

TIP

Can he O Loop? Men have tried it, but with varying degrees of success. For the average man with no difficulty getting aroused and sustaining arousal, the Orgasm Loop may just get in the way. But men who have lost their erections during lovemaking report success using the Loop. The technique is basically the same for men as it is for women: Focus on an arousal image; concentrate energy in the genitals; and use fire breathing and PC flexing (Yes, men have a PC muscle too—and using it can improve their erections and orgasms.) The goal of the O Loop is to sustain erection rather than ejaculation.

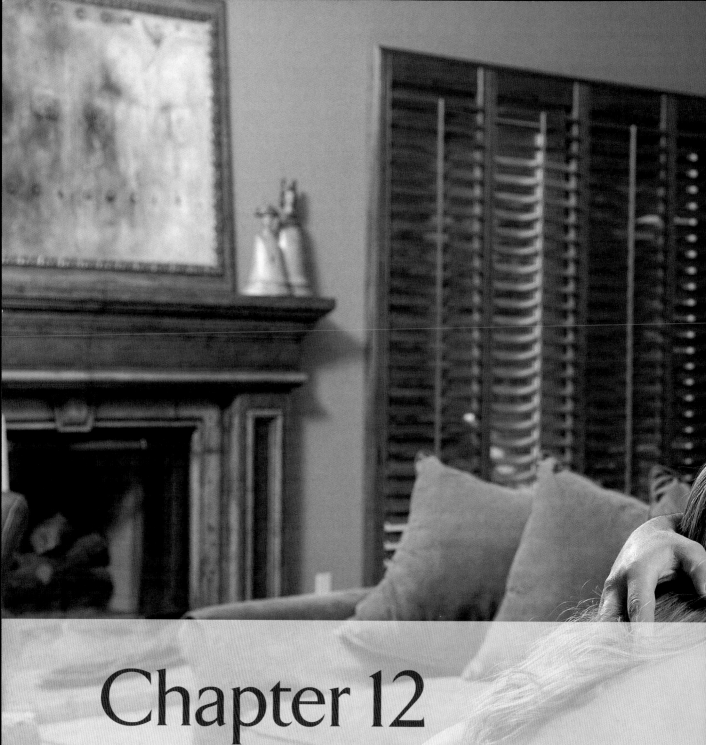

Chapter 12

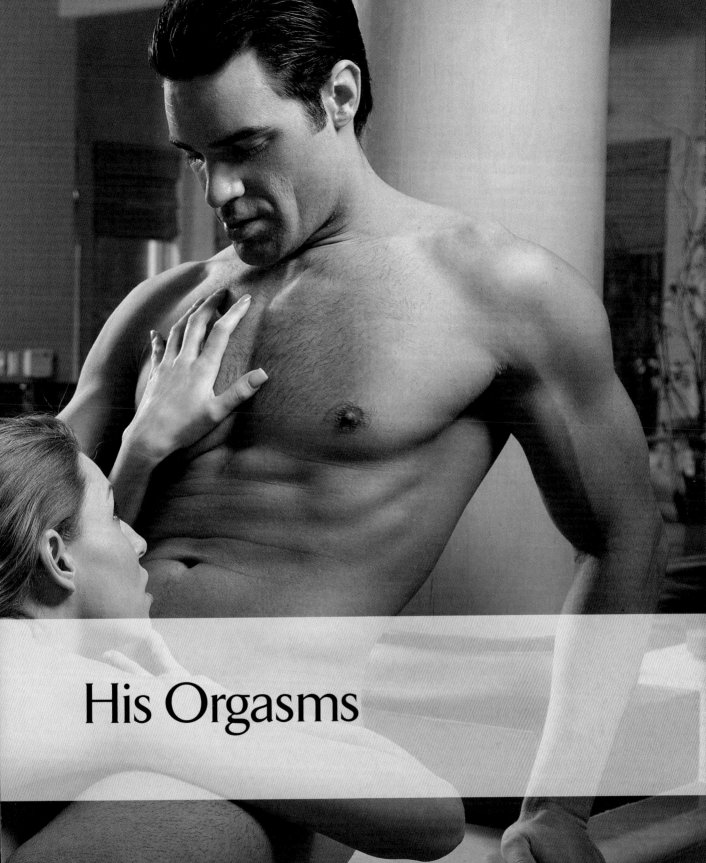

His Orgasms

The male orgasm has not received the same level of attention that the female orgasm has. Your local bookstore may have a couple dozen books on her orgasm and maybe one on his—and that will probably be a book about how he can come without ejaculating using Eastern erotic techniques. Orgasm is no problem for men, right? And one orgasm is just as good as another for him, right? And, on the other hand, he doesn't have the unlimited orgasmic potential that she has, right?

While having an orgasm may not be the issue for him as it is for her, he does experience some orgasms as "better" than others. He can learn how to have more of those if he wants to do that. And the potential for enriching his entire sexual experience through developing new orgasm skills is real.

How Does His Orgasm Differ from Hers?

Male orgasm is defined as the release of tension caused by the engorgement of blood in the genitals by contractions experienced in the penis and surrounding area, similar in timing, sequence, and length to the female orgasm. The big difference between his and hers is that the male orgasm is considered "inevitable" while the female version is described as "elusive" or "problematic."

His orgasm is "inevitable" for two reasons:

- Male masturbation is more acceptable than is female masturbation.

- Our model of partner sex is intercourse. Men reach orgasm by friction (penile thrusting) applied to the penis.

"Ejaculation is a brief episode of physical release. Orgasm is an overall feeling of intense pleasure that transcends the genital response. It is strong enough to pull down a man's emotional defenses."

—**Dr. Marty Klein**, noted therapist and author

Paths to Orgasm

While he may get there more reliably than his woman does, he doesn't have as many potential paths to ecstasy as are available to her.

Generally, men reach orgasm via stimulation of the head of the penis during intercourse or the up-and-down movement of the shaft during masturbation. There is more than one way to bring a penis to orgasm.

He can reach orgasm via:

- Fellatio (see Chapter 6 for directions)

- Manual stimulation

- Intercourse

- Anal play

- Stimulating his perineum (P zone)

As for a male G-spot, yes, he has one. See Chapter 4 for directions on how to find it.

If a man comes just by looking at a naked woman or holding and kissing her, he's fourteen (and way too young for her!) or suffers from premature ejaculation. It's a good thing if a woman can come via extra-genital stimulation, but not so good if a man does.

Thus, males orgasms are considered to be limited to three categories—ejaculatory, non-ejaculatory, and multiple—with many experts discounting the possibility of non-ejaculatory orgasm.

Can Men Have Multiples?

Whether or not men can have multiple orgasms depends largely on whether or not you accept that a man can have a non-ejaculatory orgasm. Everyone acknowledges that a man does have a refractory period after ejaculation. Some men (especially, but not only, younger men) can become erect again in a short period of time and have another ejaculatory orgasm during one lovemaking session, but this is not defined as a multiple orgasm. Sexologists are not in agreement, however, on whether or not it is possible for him to experience the contractions of orgasm without ejaculation.

The guru of self-help books and workshops on male multiples is Stan Dale, who has a doctorate in human sexuality from the Institute for the Advanced Study of Sexuality in San Francisco. According to Dale, men can learn how to experience orgasm without ejaculation. His techniques for doing that rely heavily on mental control, something men under thirty-five or forty may not have.

His main advice on the technique is to strengthen the PC muscle by doing Kegels (see Chapter 1) and to try to hold back ejaculation by using that muscle and telling yourself, "Not now, maybe later, but not now."

Repeatedly using the techniques for delaying ejaculation explained in the following section may be more effective. Some men do report that they can learn how to experience orgasmic contractions without ejaculation through repeated delaying maneuvers. Is the quest for orgasm without ejaculation worth the effort? You be the judge of that for yourself.

Delaying His Orgasm

The Eastern lovemaking arts emphasize delaying his ejaculation while intensifying her arousal. The goal is to bring her to orgasm during intercourse. As we've already figured out, he—and she—can make that happen by stimulating her clitoris. Many men do want to sustain their erections for longer periods of time during intercourse for other reasons, such as extending the pleasure for him and his partner.

The Three-Finger Draw

Practiced in China for five thousand years, this technique is simple and—men tell me—effective. Locate the midpoint of your perineum, that sensitive area between the base of the testicles and the anus. Using the three longest fingers of your right hand, apply pressure—not too light and not too hard—to this spot as soon as you feel the inevitability of orgasm. Your fingers should be curved slightly.

The trick is in finding the right spot and applying the pressure in the nick of time. That may take a little practice.

REAL TALK

Have you ever had a male G-spot orgasm?

"'Male' and 'G-spot' just shouldn't be used together like that."
—Bradley, 27

——— • ———

"Oh, yeah. I feel it in my cock and balls, my anus—
—and then it radiates throughout my pelvic area and buttocks. It's something special."
—Ryan, 41

"Dry orgasms do exist. There is documented evidence that in some cases the muscle contraction that accompanies ejaculation was not elicited by the discharge of seminal fluids."

—Prokash Kothari, M.D., international sexologist based in Mumbai, India

The Big Draw

This one requires a strong PC muscle (see Chapter 1). When you feel ejaculation is imminent, stop thrusting. Pull back to approximately 1 inch of penetration, but don't withdraw completely. Flex the PC muscle and hold to a count of nine. (Or, some men find that flexing nine times in rapid succession works better. Try it both ways.) Resume thrusting with shallow strokes.

Alternate the Stimuli

When you are highly aroused, stop thrusting and make love to your partner manually or orally. Focus on giving her pleasure. By alternating intercourse with other forms of lovemaking, most men can make the encounter last longer. In sex therapy, this is sometimes referred to as the "stop/start technique."

Count the Strokes

Based on Taoist principles, which are all about holding back ejaculation, this one is simple, but men tell me it works. Count out sets of shallow, then deep, strokes. In the classic "set of nines," a man makes nine shallow strokes (without ever withdrawing completely), then one deep one, then eight shallow strokes, then two deep ones, and so forth.

How Do You Know When His Orgasm Is Imminent?

Every man does something in exactly the same way before every orgasm. Pay attention to the subtle signs that he is close to the point of ejaculation.

For example:

- Some men hold their breath.

- Others breathe with more intensity.

- He might make a certain sound, like a grunt, cry, or exclamation, or go completely silent.

Now that you know his moment, you can spike his orgasm, or "trigger" it yourself, by:

- Stimulating his G-spot with your thumb or finger pressed gently on his perineum.

- Inserting a well-lubed finger inside his anus to stimulate the G-spot from inside, but only if he is comfortable with having that done.

Spiking His Orgasm

The emphasis is almost always on her orgasm. Will she have one? What can he do to "give" her one? How can intercourse positions be modified to help her come? But what about him? Oh, yeah, he'll come, no matter. Every now and then, let it be more about him.

If a woman thinks giving him a blow job that you finish off by swallowing is all you can do for him—and not that there's anything wrong with that—she can learn a new trick or two. Leave him gasping, leave him panting, leave him—grateful.

A simple trick for men who like to have their nipples pinched, tweaked, or bitten during foreplay is to do that at the moment of orgasm. Another easy but effective maneuver: pause. If he's on top, grab his buttocks at the moment of orgasm. Use your PC muscle to pull him in a little deeper, and make eye contact with him.

The Hip Rock 'n' Roll: Version #1: Man on Top

If he's on top and close to orgasm, grab his hip bones or buttocks and rock him, side to side or back and forth. When you control the direction of his pelvic moments, you also control the speed of thrusting and the depth of penetration. He may be on top, but you are in charge. To him, it feels like you are pulling the orgasm out of him in a very explosive way.

Do you come on her body? Does he come on your body?

"Once in a while, he does. The first time it was my idea. I said, 'I want you to come on my face,' and he was surprised but pleased. I played porn star and caught some of it my mouth and licked my lips. It's sexy. I can't explain why, but it is."
—Chantelle, 36

———•———

"I've come between my wife's breasts. She says no to the face. But maybe, one of these days . . . . It's hot to watch myself come on her breasts."
—Richard, 27

———•———

"You get the idea in the films that it is supposed to degrade the woman a little, but I like it. When he comes on my face, it's like we're doing something dirty. It's hot."
—Angela, 40

———•———

"This lady lets me do that, yes. She is the hottest woman I've ever been with. A smart, savvy businesswoman, a lady—and a tiger. She rubs my come into her nipples."
—Cornelius, 49

The Hip Rock 'n' Roll: Version #2: Woman on Top

If you're on top and he's close to orgasm, put your hands on his hips and pull him toward you. Keep your body weight on your knees so that you aren't bearing down on his hips. Again, he will feel like you're pulling that orgasm right out of him.

The Hip Rock 'n' Roll: Version #3: Fellatio

If you want to give him something really special, fellate him to orgasm. When he's near ejaculation, take his pelvis in both hands and rock him toward you so that he goes deeper into your mouth. And swallow.

The Butterfly Quiver

You'll feel like a sex goddess when you perfect this move, and it's easier than you may think it will be.

When his erection is very hard, have him slow down and let you control the thrusting dynamics of intercourse. It's easier if you're on top, but it can be done in other positions, too. His cooperation is important, because the butterfly quiver is more effective when he doesn't thrust vigorously.

Now flex your PC muscle in a continuous pattern of tightening (as you pull him inside) and releasing (as you push him out), replicating the pattern of a butterfly's pulsating wings. Make the butterfly as fast as you can when he nears ejaculation.

He will feel like his ejaculate is being pulled out of his body—a thrilling experience for both of you.

The Outside-Your-Body Experience

The "money shot" or the "cum shot" in adult films occurs when he ejaculates on her body, face and breasts being the favored targets. The popularity of that image has inspired legions of men to adapt the question "Can I come in your mouth?" into "Can I come on your face or your breasts?" It looks sexy on film. What about in real life?

Try it. You might like it. Watching a man ejaculate is both more arousing and more satisfying than you probably think it will be if you haven't done it.

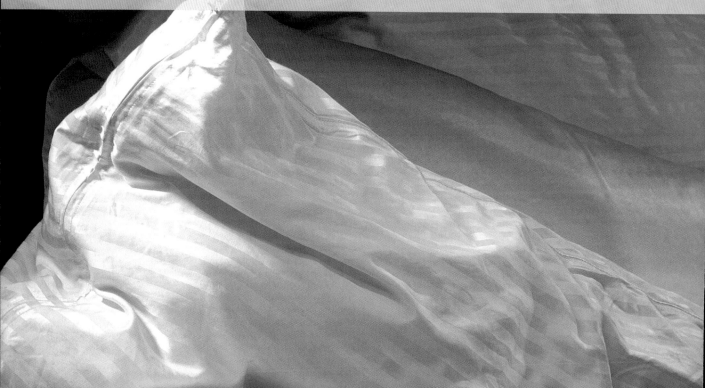

Chapter 13

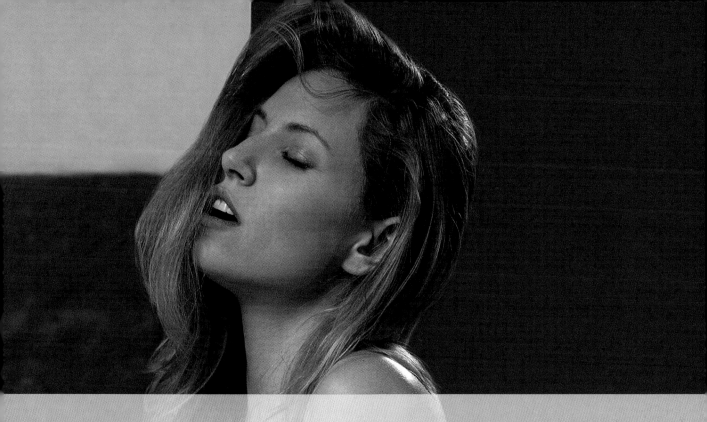

Sacred Sex: The Orgasm Connection

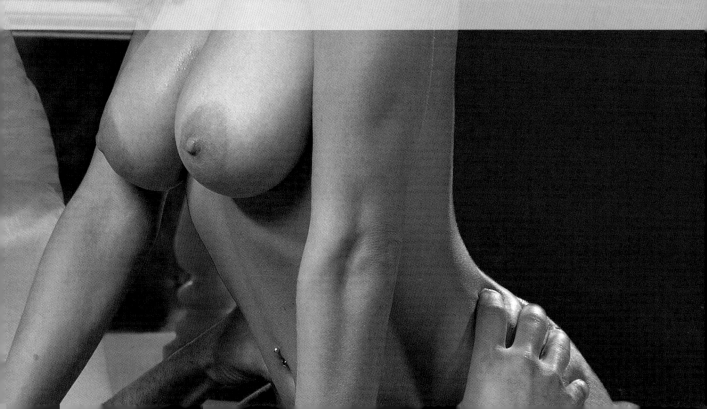

Both of you reaching orgasm during the same act of lovemaking, however it happens, makes you feel good about one another. That natural cocktail of post-orgasmic chemicals racing through your bodies enables you to gaze into your lover's eyes with renewed affection and appreciation, even if you were driving each other crazy a few hours ago. (Now that is intimacy—and you didn't have to talk about the relationship to experience it.) Orgasm smoothes the rough edges. Without good sex—and orgasm—how would men and women ever be able to live together? Or even spend a few nights a week together?

Yet some couples want to make the orgasm connection even more intense. They want simultaneous orgasms and prolonged periods of emotional as well as physical sex: sacred sex.

Simultaneous Orgasm

The simultaneous orgasm was the cultural ideal before the concept of "she comes first" took over. The old movie poster of Burt Lancaster and Deborah Kerr in *From Here to Eternity* has always symbolized that for me. Don't you think our mothers and grandmothers really believed they were coming simultaneously under those swimsuits?

While the Simultaneous O isn't quite the big deal it was back then (when she faked it in time with his), it still has a certain cachet, especially among young women who are in committed, monogamous relationships. And they do have a better chance of making that happen with their guy than single women do with casual lovers. Why?

The keys to simultaneous orgasm are communication and timing, and couples in long-term relationships are more familiar with each other's bodies and sexual responses than strangers are. You shouldn't feel pressured to make this happen, but trying to bring your orgasms together can be fun even if the timing doesn't work out.

The following three techniques may not all work for you, but they're certainly worth a try.

Stretch Out Foreplay

If you are very aroused by the foreplay (either manual, oral, or a combination) and are comfortable in giving yourself—or asking him to give you—continued manual clitoral stimulation during intercourse, you can have an intercourse orgasm fairly easily. With a little planning, you can have simultaneous orgasms. To make it happen, do the following.

Extend the warm-up. Hold off on intercourse until you are both at the "high fever" state of arousal. You know the signs: panting, sweating, flushed chest, that look in the eyes. Don't move to intercourse until you get those signals. Then move together in a state of close communication with your eyes open and your hands on each other's back, buttocks, or thighs ready to indicate "faster" or "slower." If one of you is closer to orgasm than the other, that person stops moving and signals through a sexy code phrase like "too hot" or a touch, such as gently placing your hands on the other's hips and pushing your bodies slightly away from one another.

One of the keys to simultaneous orgasm is staying connected to your lover through holding and caressing.

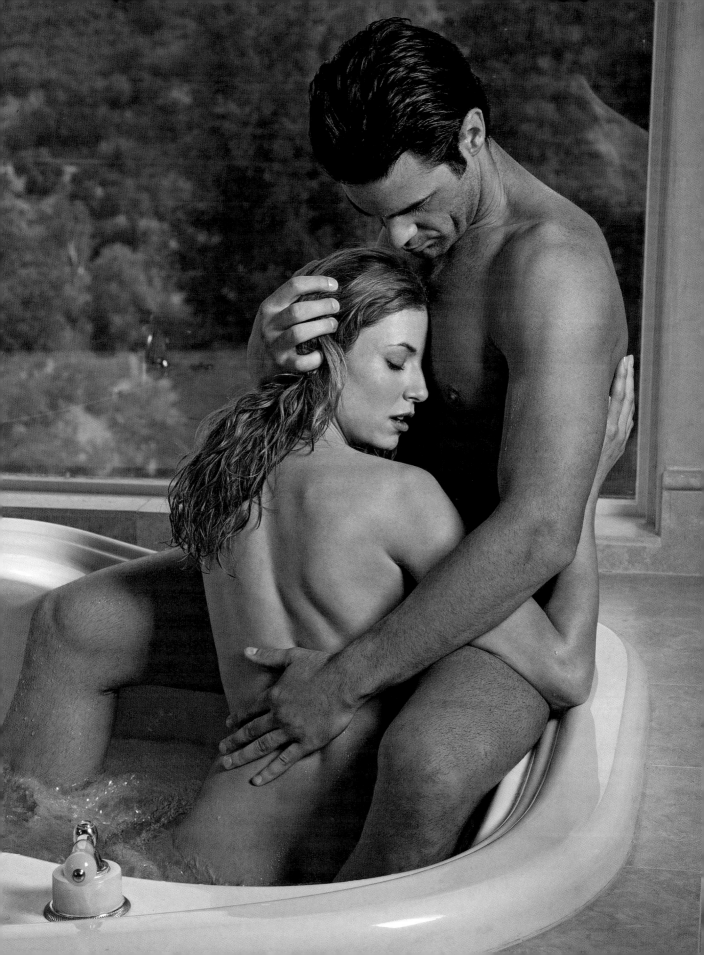

Still connected though not moving, the partner on the verge kisses, caresses, and strokes the other. Look into one another's eyes now if you are comfortable doing that, because eye contact during intercourse will let you gauge how close each other is to release, helping you time the movements. The more dilated those pupils are—that glazed and unfocused look—the closer you each are to orgasm. Now move together again to bring about simultaneous orgasms. (And you can see why only couples that know one another well can make this work.)

Why does it work? The partner who signals for a brief halt in stimulation gets the slow-down he or she needs while continuing to give the erotic attention the other needs to keep his or her arousal building. The less aroused partner continues to receive the kissing, stroking, and caressing he or she needs to catch up. This method of letting the "faster" partner focus attention on the "slower" partner until they are in sync again dramatically increases the odds that they will reach orgasm at the same time.

Forget "Ladies First"

To have a simultaneous orgasm, she should forego the prerogative of the "ladies first" orgasm through cunnilingus. Here's how to make it happen.

When he has stimulated you either orally or manually to near orgasm, pull back from the attention he is lavishing on your body by gently taking his face in your hands and pulling your hips back at the same time. As soon as you send him this physical signal, he'll understand that you

How often do you reach simultaneous orgasm with your partner?

"Almost never. But I often fake it. He loves to think that I am coming again as he is coming. It's a bit of theater I don't mind performing if I've already had mine."

—Nikki, 37

———•———

"On rare occasions—when we are really on the same page from the beginning. If I am highly aroused when we start, it is likely to happen. It is satisfying, but not necessary."

—Karen, 43

———•———

"I don't know. It seems to happen a lot, but I suspect women are faking it most of the time."

—David, 32

are ready for intercourse. He, on the other hand, may need a little extra stimulation to catch up. Ask him if he wants oral or manual pleasuring, and give him enough to bring him up to your speed. Get into the "69" position. That will give you enough additional stimulation to sustain your high while you're bringing him along. Now you're both ready!

Use eye contact to gauge each other's arousal. Also use the physical cues to control the timing—for example, grasping one another's hips to encourage faster or slower movement as needed.

This method works because, when you start intercourse at a high level of arousal, you're where he typically is at the beginning. He doesn't have to hold back.

The Adapted C.A.T. Position

The Coital Alignment Technique (C.A.T.), an adaptation of the missionary position that puts his full weight on her, has been touted as the no-fail simultaneous orgasm position. The problem? It's very uncomfortable for a woman if her partner is bigger than she is. Here's how it's done.

She lies on her back and he enters her. With his pelvis higher than hers, he lies on top of her, putting his full weight on her body. (If he's a lot taller, his chin will be resting on top of her head because he has to move his pelvis as high as it will go while sustaining the intercourse connection.) She wraps her legs around his thighs, resting her ankles on his calves. They move their pelvises only in a steady rhythm without speeding up or slowing down until they reach orgasm together.

You can adapt this basic position, taking some of the weight off her and allowing face-to-face contact, no matter your heights. While keeping your pelvises locked and her legs around his thighs as described above, he supports most of his weight on his arms. Another way to open up the C.A.T. and lift his weight off of her is for him to grasp the headboard, using that to support his weight and leverage his movements against her. Or you can reverse the C.A.T., with her on top, lying flat against him, pelvises locked, his legs wrapped around her body. In any variation, speed up or slow down that "steady rhythm" to suit your own timing needs.

This method works because the continuous stimulation this position provides your clitoris gives you the direct stimulation you need to reach orgasm during intercourse alone. Plus the constraints the position places on his movement naturally slow him down, which makes you more likely to be in sync. He moves less vigorously and at the same time gives you that steady stimulation right on target.

Achieving Sacred Sex

Sacred sex, also known as sexual ecstasy or "high sex" in some Tantric circles, is a way of making love that is supposed to incorporate body and soul in one ultimate erotic experience. Seminars and workshops on the techniques of sacred sex have proliferated in the past decade. You can book hotel getaway weekends that include afternoon classes. Bookstores devote entire sections to Tantra, the 5,000-year-old Eastern belief system that united the searches for ecstasy and enlightenment in ancient India.

The Tantric Twist

The Tantrics worshipped the god Shiva and his consort, the goddess Shakti, who they believed united the spiritual and the sexual. Their traditions included a variety of techniques then unknown in Western culture. Those traditions influenced people in other societies, including Tibet, China, and the Arab world. Eventually, they made their way West but didn't really make an impact on American society until the second half of the twentieth century.

The American way of lovemaking is goal-oriented and straightforward: Get to intercourse, orgasm, and good night. The Eastern way is about prolonging pleasure, extending orgasms, and expanding the orgasmic experience until the body seems suffused with orgasm. It's the Quickie versus the Long, Slow Love-in.

Most of us won't immerse ourselves in Tantra. (If you want to read further, the world authority on Tantra is Margot Anand, and I recommend her books because they are accessible, well written, and interesting.) We can, however, adapt some of the techniques and use them to enrich our sex lives.

Techniques for Slowing Him Down and Speeding Her Up

Tantra may be so appealing to Western lovers because it tackles the two common mind-sets that come together to create unsatisfying sex: As a boy, he learned how to masturbate quickly to avoid getting caught, while she absorbed the lesson that, for her, an orgasm wasn't nearly as important as the "feelings of closeness" generated by lovemaking. That is the basis for the kind of sex that led to the quip, "Yes, the Prince will come—too soon!"

By contrast, on the Tantric path to ecstasy, lovers are supposed to experience:

- Prolonged love play

- Prolonged intercourse

- More intense orgasms

- Longer, or extended, orgasms

- Suffused, or whole body, orgasms

- Intense emotional or spiritual connection

The techniques for making these expanded, extended, and whole body orgasms are best learned during masturbation. Expanding orgasm takes it beyond the places in the genitals where you usually experience it. Sometimes the techniques are referred to as "stretching" his orgasm and "spreading" her orgasm. If you master these techniques, they simply make your orgasm feel a little more diffuse, bathing the genitals and immediately beyond in pleasure. And they feel stronger.

Expanding Orgasm, Hers

Using your fingers or a vibrator, masturbate in a comfortable position. As soon as you become highly aroused, use one hand to massage with light, shallow strokes the area of your vulva, inner thighs, and groin. Imagine that you are spreading your arousal throughout those areas. Continue the massage throughout your orgasm, imagining you are spreading your orgasm into your body.

After orgasm, continue rhythmic stroking of your genital area. Feel the orgasm continuing to spread throughout your body for several seconds after it normally would have dissipated.

Expanding Orgasm, His

Masturbate without ejaculating for as long as you can. (A reasonable goal is ten to fifteen minutes, though maybe not the first time.) Do this by stopping and/or changing strokes when ejaculation is imminent.

Count the contractions you feel upon ejaculation, normally between three and eight. Note the level and order of intensity. Typically the strongest contractions will be at the beginning. The next time you masturbate, again delay ejaculation as long as possible.

When you do ejaculate, flex your PC muscle as you would to retard ejaculation. Then continue stimulating your penis very slowly while squeezing throughout the ejaculation, thus pushing the sensations on and on.

Staying on the Edge

Now that you have learned how to expand orgasm, extending—or making it last longer—is a fairly easy step up to the next level of "high sex." This is a couple's game. Take a cool, not hot, shower together. Your skin should be cool to the other's touch as you begin.

Lie on the bed side by side, facing one another, with your legs entwined in a scissors position. Insert his flaccid penis into her vagina. Both remain still. One of you may have to keep a hand around the base of his penis to keep it inside until he has a moderate erection. (But don't work to make him have one!)

Breathing deeply, try to remain motionless for 15 to 30 minutes. During this time, caress each other's faces, necks, and upper bodies, and make frequent, prolonged eye contact. Whisper terms of endearment. Are you feeling a sense of erotic peace?

Now begin moving together. He should be thrusting slowly and gently and she should be matching his pace with her pelvis and hips. Kiss deeply. As you move your bodies, use your hands to stroke each other, working upward from one another's genitals. Imagine that you are spreading fire with your hands.

Resist the desire to move faster when you reach that agonizing point of being "almost there." You want to stay on the verge for as long as possible—until you realize that you are having an orgasm. It will seem to last forever.

More Games for Experienced Lovers

You can expand and extend? Are you ready to take it even higher?

Karezza

An Italian word that means "caress," Karezza was developed by an American physician in 1883. Alice Bunker Stockholm borrowed it in part from a pamphlet on birth control written by a founding member of the Oneida community, a minister who adapted it from the ancient erotic teachings of a Chinese physician named Master Sun. Stockholm instructed her married patients in the art of Karezza as a way to prevent his premature ejaculation while allowing sufficient time for her arousal. Her small self-published book, *Karezza: Ethics of Marriage*, was translated into several languages, including Russian by the great novelist Leo Tolstoy.

In her book she instructed readers to remain in a sexual position for an hour without moving toward orgasm. And she encouraged them to read aloud from Ralph Waldo Emerson and Elizabeth Barrett Browning, and then discuss the meaning of those works. That is one of the most interesting pieces of erotic history I've ever uncovered.

As a technique for prolonging intercourse, Karezza is simple and effective and can be practiced in any position. It also encourages extended orgasm.

Any intercourse position can work, but man-on-top or missionary is least likely to encourage Karezza. Woman-on-top or female superior and side-by-side are better choices. The key is to dramatically limit his genital movement. He does not move inside the woman unless he becomes flaccid. Then he takes only shallow strokes to revive his erection.

"People who come into sex therapy have basic problems. They just want to have sex occasionally and they certainly aren't asking how to make good sex great. People go to the bookstores for that. The average sex therapist couldn't tell a couple how to perform Karezza if her fee depended on it."

—X, a famous sex therapist and author

Couples can also try Karezza in the standing position. The male should stay as still as possible while the woman moves in whatever way best stimulates her own orgasm.

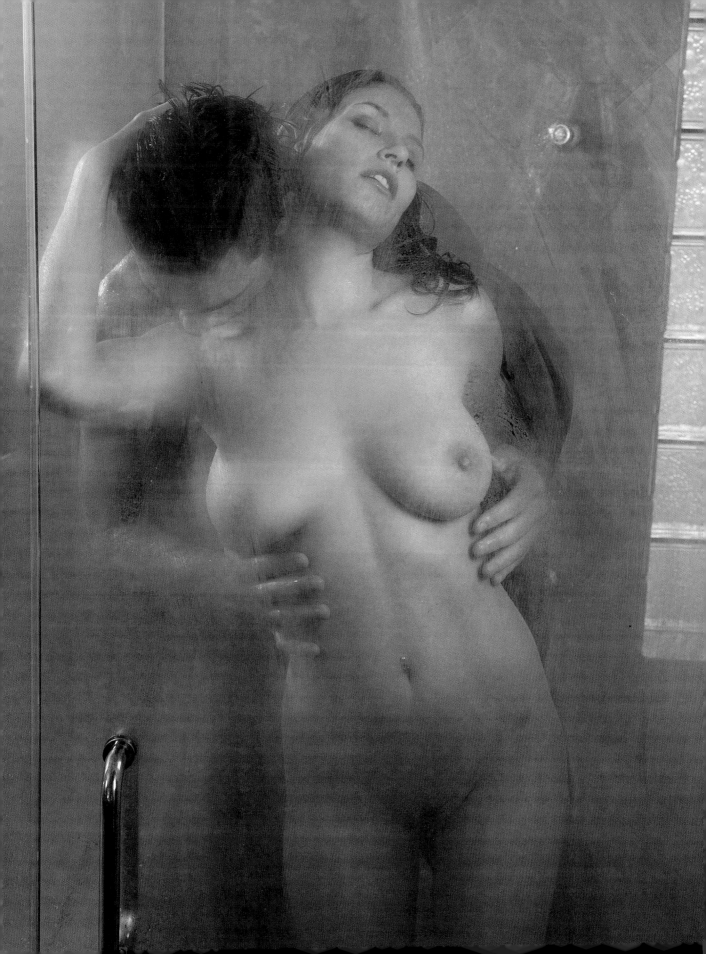

She is allowed to move, including thrusting her hips against his and contracting her PC muscle around his penis. No matter how excited she gets, he takes only sufficient thrusting strokes to maintain an erection. Using the masturbation technique of expanding or "spreading," she (or he) encourages the spread of her orgasm throughout her body.

He holds their lovemaking embrace until she has had one or several orgasms. Then he is free to move with more energy and satisfy himself.

Kabbazah

Now it's his turn to be intensely pleasured.

I first heard about Kabbazah while interviewing a man for a story in *Penthouse Forum* magazine many years ago. He'd received the sex experience of his life in Japan as a soldier on R&R leave from Vietnam. "I paid three times the going rate for it," he said, "and that was a bargain."

Kabbazah was actually developed thousands of years ago in the Middle East, when religious extremists did not dominate that part of the world. A woman who had mastered the French art of pompoir (control of the PC muscle) was called a kabbazah, or "one who holds." Kabbazahs included the best prostitutes in many Eastern countries, including China, Japan, and India. Prostitution was sacred in India, and the temple prostitutes believed that they brought a man to religious as well as sexual ecstasy via Kabbazah. The lifestyle of these upper level Eastern prostitutes was the equivalent of that enjoyed by today's most expensive international call girls.

As I researched Kabbazah, Karezza, and other techniques, I was struck by how sexologists in the late twentieth century, such as the famed Mumbai sexologist Dr. Prokash Kothari, were developing theories and techniques similar to those of ancient times. A really good idea never dies. And Kabbazah is a good idea.

There are two absolute requirements for its practice:

- He must be in a relaxed and receptive state of mind and body. His passivity is crucial. This is not the kind of sex you have when you are desperately tearing each other's clothing off.

- She must have a virtuoso vagina. Don't even try this until you have diligently practiced Kegels for a period of three weeks to a month.

Here's how the technique works. Begin in the female superior or sitting intercourse position. She stimulates her partner until he is just erect, not highly aroused. Now she inserts his penis.

He does not move his pelvis at all. Not once. She also strives for no pelvic movement, confining all movements—or as much as possible—to her PC muscle. You may, however, caress and kiss each other.

She flexes her muscle in varying patterns until she feels his penis throbbing, which should occur approximately fifteen minutes into Kabbazah. At that point, he should be highly aroused. She times her contractions to the throbbing of his penis, clenching and releasing in time with him.

In another ten to fifteen minutes, he will experience a longer, more intense orgasm than normal.

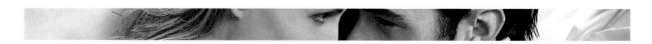

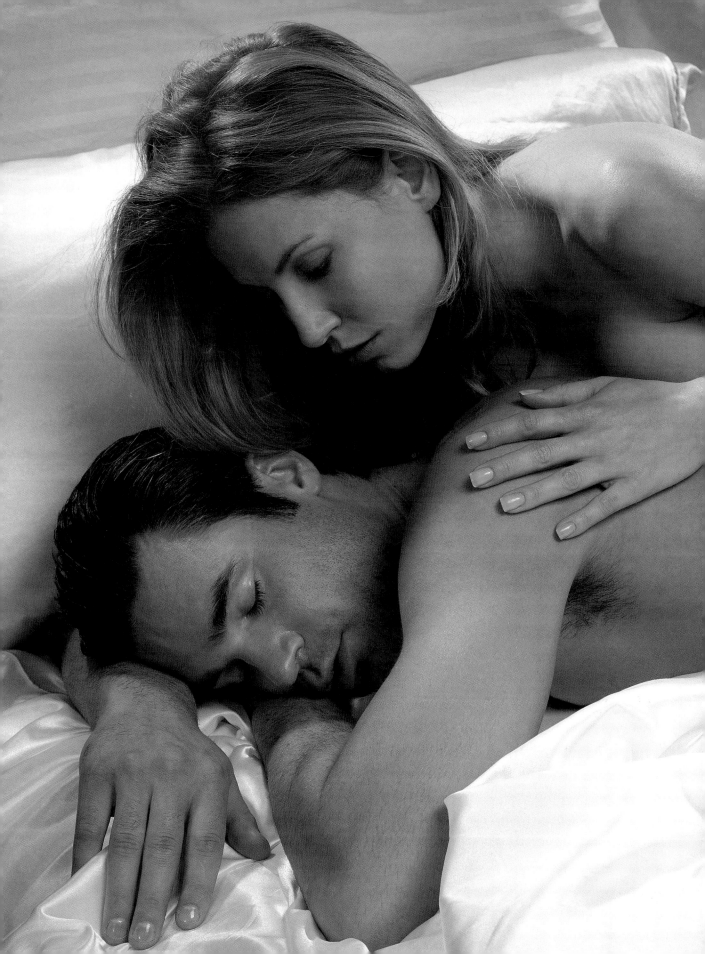

Whole Body Orgasm

Have you ever heard someone say, "I felt that orgasm all the way down to my toes"? Or, "My orgasm almost blew the top of my head off"? Maybe you've even said something like this yourself.

When you experience an orgasm that is clearly an event taking place beyond your genitals, you're having a whole body orgasm. Some people see flashing lights or colors. Others say it feels like an out-of-body experience. Many describe feeling a strong, emotional connection to their partners.

The whole body orgasm is most likely the result of intense connections on three levels: emotional, sensual, and sexual. Consider the levels to be separate doors, three ways into the whole body orgasm.

Emotional: The Tantric Kiss

Some proponents of Kundalini (or sexual) yoga say that its practice encourages stronger emotional connections between partners. Certainly there are Kundalini techniques designed to promote an emotional as well as a physical closeness between lovers. The kiss is particularly intimate and sacred in Tantra.

During the kiss, the soul and energy of one partner is thought to flow into the other, and vice versa. This dovetails nicely with the Western concept of being "soul mate" partners. That may be too esoteric for most of us, but who doesn't get into a deep, soulful kiss now and again? To practice the Tantric yoga kiss, do the following.

During intercourse (in any position), he practices one of the methods described earlier in this chapter to delay his orgasm and ejaculation. When she feels her own orgasm is imminent, she signals him to stop moving. The couple sits in the middle of the bed with his penis inside her, legs wrapped around each other, moving as little as possible.

Pressing your foreheads together, breathe into each other's mouths. As he exhales, she inhales. And vice versa. Prolong this "kiss" until remaining still is no longer an option. Movement will trigger orgasm. The long, slow arousal period and the emotional intensity of the kiss can combine to make your orgasm feel like a whole body experience.

Sensual: Extra-Genital Orgasm

For some people, especially women, the whole body orgasm is not the first orgasm during a lovemaking session. If she's already had one or more orgasms, she may be ready to experience extra-genital orgasm. She's on a sensual high. With the right touch, she could take it even higher. Here's how.

After she's had at least one orgasm, caress her vagina and perform cunnilingus if she requests it. When she is on the verge of another orgasm, move your hands and mouth away from her genitals. Stroke her breasts, nipples, inner thighs—whatever non-genital area she wants touched, kissed, or licked. She may be in such a state of hypersensitivity that she reaches orgasm this way, and the orgasm will feel like it is spread throughout her body.

If not, stimulate her clitoris orally or manually as you continue to pay attention to non-genital areas. (To a purist, this might be "cheating," but who cares?)

Sexual: The Yabyum and Passion Flower

For some people, a whole body orgasm happens when the sex is more intense than usual. It's not about the emotions and sensuality, at least not until the afterglow sets in. The sex—down and dirty, hard and fast, hot and hotter—is what takes them to the place where they can savor the sensual, the place where their guard is finally down and they can feel the emotions. If you are that person or your lover is, open your bag of sex tricks now.

The Yabyum, a Tantric version of the Western sitting position, is a must-try. It is highly touted by sexologists as the ultimate position for prolonging male arousal and intensifying lovers' intimate connection. You will like it, even if you are not all that turned on by Tantra. The Yabyum: Sit in the center of the bed facing each other. Wrap your legs around one another so she is sitting on his thighs. Place your right hands at the back of each other's neck, your left hands on each other's tailbones. Now stroke each other's back, using upward strokes only. Look deeply into one another's eyes as you kiss with eyes open.

Put his semi-erect penis inside her vagina so it exerts as much indirect pressure as possible on her clitoris and makes G-spot contact. (She can sit on pillows rather than his thighs, if necessary, to get the angle of penetration right.)

Perform the Tantric kiss described earlier in this chapter. Rock slowly together while continuing to rub each other's back and sustaining deep eye contact. Maintain this position until both orgasm. This is the Yabyum.

Several years ago the editors of *Redbook* magazine asked me to develop a new sex position for their readers—a position that addressed some common concerns and complaints.

The position had to:

- Give her maximum clitoral and/or G-spot stimulation during intercourse

- Enable him to be highly aroused yet sustain intercourse longer than usual

- Give them both exceptional orgasms

- Provide the feeling of greater intimacy than the average intercourse position

The Yabyum came immediately to mind. But I wanted something a little less time-consuming and easier for couples that might not be yoga devotees to do. Why not start in the Yabyum—a looser version, essentially used as intense foreplay—and then open it up, like a flower unfolding? The resulting position, The Passion Flower, was a hit with testers and later with readers, too.

The Passion Flower: As in the Yabyum, start in the center of the bed, facing one another. Wrap her legs comfortably around his body. She may either sit on his thighs or on pillows positioned in front of him. Her legs can be splayed out straight or bent at the knees, whichever is more comfortable for him.

Place your right hands on each other's neck and your left hands at the base of each other's spine. Stroke each other's back, using upward strokes only. Look into each other's eyes and kiss with eyes open. Continue kissing and stroking until you're both highly aroused.

Insert his erect penis into her vagina so that the shaft exerts as much indirect pressure on her clitoris as possible. Rock together, slowly rubbing each other's backs and kissing deeply. She may reach orgasm quickly in this position. After her first orgasm (or sooner, if she doesn't feel orgasm is imminent) move into one of the following variations:

He sits on the bed with his legs open wide. She lies back on the bed, facing him, with her body between his legs. He lifts her ankles up against his shoulders and enters her at a comfortable angle. She keeps her thighs closed, creating a tighter grip on his penis. And she uses one hand to stimulate her clitoris.

She lies on her back, again between his legs, but with her legs bent at the knees and pulled back against her body until her heels touch her thighs. He sits close to her with his penis opposite her vagina. She places her knees under his armpits and has him gently pull closer until he can comfortably insert his penis. Again, she stimulates her clitoris during thrusting.

TIP

——— • ———

Keeping your eyes open during kissing and intercourse is not a one-size-fits-all erotic technique. Some couples find the deep soul-gazing intrusive or even silly. Don't be dogmatic about open eyes—or anything else, for that matter. If you are more comfortable making love with your eyes closed, go with what feels good to you. Do try opening your eyes occasionally to make eye contact with your lover, though.

Are You There Yet?

I know that, if you are reading these words, you are having better orgasms than you were having when you opened this book. If something wasn't happening for you within these pages, you would have tossed the book aside many hours ago. You are, as a Yogi master I know is fond of saying, finding your bliss.

Stay on that path. The more satisfying sex you have, the more you want. Use this book like a cookbook. Keep returning to it for gourmet orgasm recipes. And lest you think I put all my faith in technique and none in passion, let me close with some of my favorite words from Anaïs Nin, the erotic diarist whose life and work celebrated passion.

"Sex loses all its power and magic when it becomes explicit, mechanical, overdone, when it becomes a mechanistic obsession. It is wrong not to mix sex with emotion, hunger, desire, lust, whims, caprices, personal ties, deeper relationships that change its color, flavor, rhythms ..."

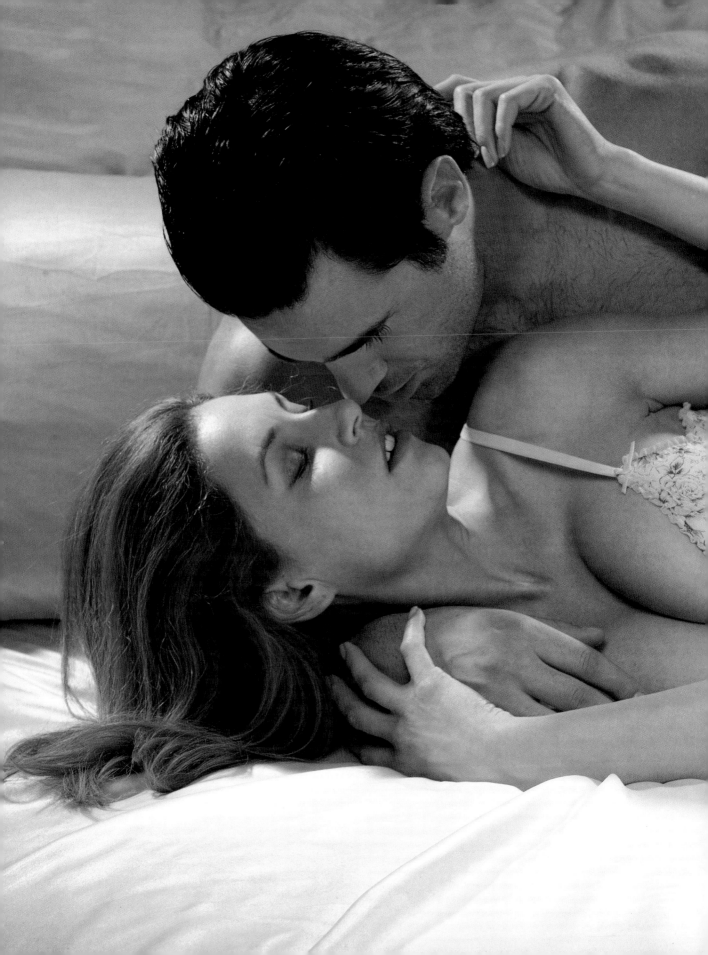

Acknowledgments

As always, thank you first and foremost to Richard Curtis, my agent.

Thanks also to:

Professional colleagues who inspire and encourage: Dr. Patti Britton, Dr. Bob Berkowitz, Dr. Barry Komisaruk—and the bright, cheeky Babes who write about sex: Lou Paget, Carlin Ross, Tracy Cox, Susie Bright, and Tristan Taormino.

My editors Wendy Gardner and Jill Alexander, project manager Amanda Waddell, copy editor Karen Levy, publisher Will Kiester, creative director Rosalind Wanke, and the amazing design team at Quiver.

My friends and family who have lent support and encouragement over the years, especially Carolyn Males, Michael and Barb Hasamear, Alex Zola, Joe Rinaldi . . . and my DIL Tammy Bakos who has given us the incomparable Marcella and delightful twin boys.

New friends in the 'hood, Elizabeth, Corey, and Reggie—what would I have done without you?

Adam & Eve, Babeland, and Candida Royalle for providing a wealth of free sex toys used in research of this book.

And especially to my collaborators—models Jamie Lynn and Charles Dera—for making this book elegant and erotic.

INDEX